Drugs that Don't Work *and*
NATURAL THERAPIES THAT DO!

2nd Edition

David Brownstein, M.D.

For further copies of ***Drugs That Don't Work and Natural Therapies That Do, 2nd Edition:***

Call: **1-888-647-5616** or send a check or money order in the amount of: $20.00 ($15.00 plus $5.00 shipping and handling) or for Michigan residents $20.90 ($15.00 plus $5.00 shipping and handling, plus $.90 sales tax) to:

Medical Alternatives Press
4173 Fieldbrook
West Bloomfield, Michigan 48323

Drugs That Don't Work and Natural Therapies That Do, 2nd Edition:
Copyright © 2009 by David Brownstein, M.D.
All Rights Reserved
No part of this book may be reproduced without written consent from the publisher.

ISBN: 978-0-9660882-6-7
Medical Alternatives Press
4173 Fieldbrook
West Bloomfield, Michigan 48323
(248) 851-3372
(888) 647-5616

Acknowledgements

I gratefully acknowledge the help I have received from my friends and colleagues in putting this book together. This book could not have been published without help from the editors—my wife Allison, Tracey Hartlieb, Dr. Guy Abraham, Janet Darnell, Mary Ann Block, Dr. Rob Radtke, and my partners Dr. Rick Ng and Dr. Jeff Nusbaum.

I would also like to thank my patients. It is your search for safe and effective natural treatments that is the driving force behind holistic medicine. You have accompanied me down this path and I appreciate each and every one of you.

And, to my staff. Thank you so very much for taking this trip with me. Without your help and support, none of this would be possible. I do appreciate all of your hard work and your dedication.

A Word of Caution to the Reader

The information presented in this book is based on the training and professional experience of the author. The treatments recommended in this book should not be undertaken without first consulting a physician. Proper laboratory and clinical monitoring is essential to achieving the goals of finding safe and natural treatments. This book was written for informational and educational purposes only. It is not intended to be used as medical advice.

ABOUT THE AUTHOR

David Brownstein, M.D. is a family physician who utilizes the best of conventional and alternative therapies. He is the Medical Director for the Center for Holistic Medicine in West Bloomfield, MI. Dr. Brownstein is a graduate of the University of Michigan and Wayne State University School of Medicine. He is Board-Certified by The American Academy of Family Practice. Dr. Brownstein is a member of the American Academy of Family Physicians and the American College for the Advancement in Medicine. He is the father of two wonderful girls, Hailey and Jessica. Dr. Brownstein has lectured internationally about his success using natural items. Dr. Brownstein has authored nine books: _The Miracle of Natural Hormones 3rd Edition, Overcoming Thyroid Disorders 2nd Edition, Overcoming Arthritis, Iodine: Why You Need It, Why You Can't Live Without It 4th Edition, The Guide to Healthy Eating, Salt Your Way to Health, The Guide to a Gluten-Free Diet,_ and _The Guide to a Dairy-Free Diet._

Dr. Brownstein's office is located at:

Center for Holistic Medicine
5821 W. Maple Rd.
Ste. 192
West Bloomfield, MI 48323
248.851.1600
www.drbrownstein.com
www.centerforholisticmedicine.com

Contents

Foreword   8

Chapter 1:   Introduction   13

Chapter 2:   Cholesterol-Lowering Drugs   25

Chapter 3:   New Studies on Cholesterol-Lowering Drugs   61

Chapter 4:   Diabetes Drugs   73

Chapter 5:   Osteoporosis Drugs   101

Chapter 6:   Antacid Drugs   157

Chapter 7:   Antidepressant Drugs   197

Chapter 8:   Anti-inflammatory Drugs   239

Chapter 9:   Hormone Replacement Therapy   275

Final Thoughts   297

Index: 304

DEDICATION

To the women of my life: Allison, Hailey and Jessica, with all my love

To my patients who seek out safe and effective treatments

To my staff, who are some of the most dedicated people I have ever worked with

FOREWORD

Some aspects of medicine and health care have made enormous progress over the last 100 years. Surgical improvements and innovations have enabled life-saving procedures not even imagined a century ago. Much more accurate diagnoses are possible with modern diagnostic equipment. Emergency medicine and trauma care in 2009 is vastly superior to that of even three or four decades ago.

But there's one aspect of medicine where very little—if any—overall progress has been made since the very early 1900s. In this part of medicine, it's time to recognize the problem, and simply start over again.

What part of medicine is this? It's the entire field of "drug therapy". For 100 years, mainstream medicine has been "spinning its wheels" while using drug therapy to suppress symptoms, but making very little genuine progress towards real health improvement.

How can this be? Aren't modern drugs the best therapy ever? We're constantly bombarded with propaganda telling us of the wonders of the most recently "approved" drugs (frequently followed a few years later by exposés of the initially well hidden, often lethal hazards of these same drugs), but we're not ever told that the entire concept of "drug therapy" is a blind alley, a dead-end road, a century-old illusion.

Using drugs and expecting them to truly improve the long-term function of your body is like putting water, alcohol, orange juice, or any other liquid except motor oil into your car's engine, and expecting it to work smoothly for as long as it would with motor oil. Your car's engine is not designed to work for it's intended lifetime with anything except motor oil, and your body is not designed to work for it's lifetime with drugs in it.

What are 21st century "therapeutic drugs", anyway? At present, and for the last 100 years, almost all therapeutic drugs have been patented molecules. (In the 19th century, this sort of drug was called a "patent medication", and routinely ridiculed.) Since the law says that only molecules *never* found in human bodies or in Nature can be patented, drugs—patent medicines—must be molecules never, ever naturally found in you or me or Nature or even on planet Earth!

Think about that. It means that for the last 100 years or so, mainstream medicine has been trying to improve your health and mine using—literally speaking—extraterrestrial molecules, molecules never before seen on planet Earth!

Please don't misunderstand. I'm not "going off the deep end" about little green men and other space aliens. Those beings, if they exist at all, are not running the companies which make enormous profits from patent medications or 'approved drugs'.

How can molecules never before found on planet Earth possibly be good for your body or mine? The molecules from which our bodies are made—except for basic elements like hydrogen, carbon, and oxygen, found throughout the Universe—are 100% of Earthly origin.

Like engines designed to run long and smoothly using motor oil, our bodies are designed to live long and healthy made up and fueled by molecules naturally found in human bodies or at least from planet Earth!

Unfortunately, "mainstream medicine" has been trying to improve the health of Earthly, human bodies by using molecules never found in human bodies or on our planet for approximately the last 100 years.

It's time to start over again, this time with natural medicine, which works with molecules found in our bodies or in Nature—amino acids, essential fatty acids, vitamins, minerals, botanicals, and many others— which actually help our bodies repair themselves as bodies are designed to do, rather than just suppressing symptoms. The natural approach (also called "alternative", "holistic", "complementary", and "integrative" medicine) works with the substances of which our bodies are made. What could be more logical? And as Dr. Brownstein writes, it's also very effective, and much safer than those "extraterrestrial" drugs!

In the early 1980s, I started working with "bio-identical hormones", hormones exactly, precisely identical to those found naturally in women's and men's bodies. I wrote the very first prescriptions in North Amerca (sourced and filled by pharmacist Ed Thorpe of Kripps Pharmacy, Vancouver, British Columbia) for bio-identical estrogen replacement for women, and combined them with bio-identical progesterone, testosterone, and DHEA. I copied Nature (and hundreds of thousands of years of human hormonal function) in every way possible: identical molecules, in quantities naturally found in human bodies (no more, no less), timing their use to mimic Nature, and copying Nature's pathways of introduction into the body. The women (and fewer numbers of men) I worked with told me over and over "I feel like myself again".

But for years, I was told by mainstream doctors and professors that using exact duplicates of Nature's hormones was "unproven" and "had unknown dangers". Mainstream medicine had women take patented extraterrestrial molecules called "progestins", along with horse hormones (at least from this planet, but over 70% never before found in women's bodies)—deliberately misnamed "HRT", hormone replacement therapy—and said it was "well-studied", "proven" and "the consensus".

Well, we all know what's happened to HRT. When actually studied ("Women's Health Initiative"), it was found dangerous. The patented, extraterrestrial "progestins" (as anyone but "mainstream medicine" would predict) were found more even more hazardous than the also dangerous, 70% not found in women, but still naturally-occurring horse estrogens.

While I'm no longer hearing that "HRT" is well studied, proven, and the consensus, it probably is no surprise that "mainstream" physicians and professors still refuse to consider that long-term drug therapy (patent medicine therapeutics—extraterrestrial molecules) are almost entirely a dead-end road. They're still telling me (and you) that copying hundreds of thousands of years of natural hormone function in women and men is "unproven" and "risky".

In this book, Dr. David Brownstein gives us example after example of the dead-end road of patent medication use, with its inevitable health-damaging effects. Even better, he outlines Nature's alternatives; amino acids to rebuild levels of serotonin and other neurotransmitters instead of using "extraterrestrial molecules" (patented drug therapy) to artificially prop them up; minerals, vitamins, and bio-identical hormones to build and maintain healthy bones instead of yet another extraterrestrial molecule to literally poison a whole category of bone cells; and many, many other ways to improve your health by following Nature's plan.

I'm always pleased when Dr. Brownstein asks me to write a foreword for one of his many books because I know I'll be impressed and learn something. Once again I have.

I'm also impressed by his courage and true dedication to his patients' health. Despite his medical education, which like mine emphasized the use of patent medications--extraterrestrial molecules— Dr. Brownstein observed his patients closely, saw they weren't doing well, found Nature's way, and then acted on it. Given the political power of "organized medicine" that takes courage.

Dr. Brownstein is one of a slowly growing minority of physicians who recognize that human bodies are natural systems, which when ill are best served by natural remedies. Of course there are always a few exceptions, usually emergencies, but for most circumstances, medicine and health care must replace the dead-end of "drug therapy" with Nature's molecules following Nature's patterns.

Technology in medicine is truly wonderful, and here to stay. Physicians practicing natural medicine use it whenever appropriate and necessary. But it's well past time for *all* of medicine to recognize that helping human bodies to truly heal and stay healthy, we should first use molecules naturally present in human bodies. "Extraterrestrial" patent medicines—"drug therapy" should be used rarely and only if the natural approach fails.

As written many centuries ago:

"Natural forces are the healers of disease."

---Hippocrates (~460-377 B.C.)

"The physician is only the servant of Nature, not her master. Therefore it behooves medicine to follow the will of nature."

----Paracelsus (1493-1541)

---Jonathan V. Wright, M.D.
Tahoma Clinic, Renton, Washington

Author: ***Book of Nutritonal Therapy*** (1978)
Guide to Healing with Nutrition (1984)
with Lane Lenard, Ph.D.:
Natural Hormone Replacement for Women over 45 (1997)
Why Stomach Acid is Good For You (2001)
With Alan R.Gaby, M.D.
Natural Medicine, Optimal Wellness (2006)

Chapter 1

Introduction

INTRODUCTION

It has been over two years since I wrote the first edition of Drugs That Don't Work and Natural Therapies That Do. Since that time the research about the most commonly used drug therapies has strengthened my opinions. This new edition of this book will show you why you need to seek safe and effective natural therapies and try to avoid life-long prescription drug use.

The latest cholesterol research—The JUPITOR and ENHANCE Studies certainly continue to call into question the cholesterol=heart disease hypothesis. These studies, and others, are reviewed in chapter 3.

The epidemic of diabetes is upon us. Americans are the most obese people on the planet and suffering from diabetes at record levels. In chapter 4 I discuss the conventional approaches to diabetes and the problems with using the oral type 2 diabetic medications. Diabetes is a lifestyle illness and can be corrected by treating the underlying cause—poor lifestyle choices. I fear that if we don't change our ways, our standard of living will begin to decline due to the diabetic epidemic that has begun.

All of the information in this book can be summed up by one statement; *you can't poison a crucial enzyme or block an important receptor for the long-term and expect a good result.* This statement forms the basis of my belief that the long-term use of many drug therapies are often harmful for the body and should be used as a last resort or for a short course of emergent treatment.

I am a conventionally trained, board-certified family practitioner. Becoming a family physician was my lifelong dream. I completed medical school and a residency in family practice and began practicing what I was taught—conventional medicine. In other words, I was an expert in prescribing a multitude of drugs to treat a variety of conditions.

I fully bought into the concept that once an appropriate diagnosis was made, there was a drug available to treat the illness. I received and read the medical journals that were pertinent to my specialty. Nearly all of the articles were showing positive results with a particular drug to treat a condition. In fact, it was rare to see a negative article about a drug. I would be visited by many pharmaceutical representatives who would show me fancy brochures on the latest studies about the drugs they were promoting. I went to many lunches and dinners where speakers showed me the research that the so-called drug of the day was the best thing for my patients.

During this time, I was prescribing these wonder drugs to my patients. It was almost expected at the office visit that a drug would be prescribed. If a patient had a chronic illness, they were usually on a combination of drugs. However, after a short period of time, this type of medicine did not sit right with me.

In fact, I began to get an uneasy feeling about what I was doing. I realized that I was medicating nearly all of my patients with drugs that were only treating the symptoms of their illness. These drugs were not addressing the underlying causes of the patients' illnesses. Furthermore, there were a significant amount of adverse effects from these drugs. I was not observing the improvement of my patients' health with the use of these drugs. Over time, I began to have trouble sleeping at night as I was thinking about how many drugs I was prescribing.

The number of sleepless nights increased until I had to tell my wife, out of the blue, that I did not want to be a doctor anymore. I became unhappy with the drug-prescribing approach to the practice of medicine. I felt that I was treating patients with one drug after another that, most of the time, did not treat the underlying cause of the illness. Furthermore, these drugs were causing many side effects, for which I prescribed more drugs. I was treating the drug side effects with more medications!

I began to realize that I was not helping my patients treat the underlying causes of their illnesses, nor was I helping them become healthy. In fact, I did not know how to achieve these results. I was not taught in medical school about what health is and how to maintain it. I was taught about pathology and the diagnosis of illness and how to treat the illness through a drug therapy.

I took an oath in medical school that said in part, "Above all, do no harm." As I began to take a closer look at the drugs I was prescribing, my uneasiness worsened. Using the physiology and biochemistry that I learned in medical school, I became more and more aware of the risks and adverse effects that accompany the long-term use of many commonly prescribed drugs. It was at this point in my career that I began to search for another way to treat my patients.

I started on a search for a less toxic approach to helping my patients not only overcome an illness but to achieve their optimal health. I began looking at lifestyle changes, including dietary changes. I began investigating the use of natural agents such as vitamins, minerals, herbs, and bioidentical hormones for treating illnesses as well as promoting health.

MY FATHER'S STORY

My father was my first test case. He had suffered from severe coronary artery disease since the age of 40, when he had his first heart attack. He had continual angina for over 20 years as well as a cholesterol level well over 300mg/dl. My father was seeing the best doctors around and he was being treated with a number of medications to control his blood pressure, blood sugar and cholesterol.

My father felt terrible. He had no energy. He could not do anything, as he would get angina at the slightest activity. He had a pasty appearance and he looked as if he was going to die.

A chiropractor (Robert Radtke, D.C.) gave me a book, **_Healing with Nutrition,_** by Jonathan Wright, M.D. Dr. Wright wrote about his success with many different natural items in treating numerous conditions. I focused on the chapter that discussed heart disease. Dr. Wright wrote about his success in using natural therapies to treat as well as prevent illness. I had my father come into the office and, after testing, I prescribed a course of therapy that included the use of natural, bioidentical hormones as well as vitamins and minerals (Vitamin C and magnesium).

The results were astounding. Within one week, his angina was gone. Within four weeks, his cholesterol level fell below 200mg/dl for the first time in years. My father was able to come off of cholesterol lowering medications without changing his diet (much to my consternation). He lost weight. He lost the pasty color to his face and he no longer looked as if he was going to die. This all occurred with therapies that were not taught to me in my medical training. When I saw the changes in my father, I knew this was the type of medicine I would pursue for the future.

From that moment on, I began to research the use of natural items to not only treat illness, but to promote health. ***Natural items generally do not poison crucial enzymes or block important receptors.*** Because our bodies have receptors for natural items, these items have few adverse side effects when used appropriately. Unlike most drug therapies, natural therapies generally do not stay in the body for a prolonged period of time. It is much more difficult for the body to detoxify a drug as compared to a vitamin or mineral therapy.

In medical school we studied a tremendous amount of biochemistry. It was tedious work memorizing how biochemical pathways worked. Furthermore, we learned which substances blocked these pathways and which items stimulated them. Drugs, being foreign substances to the body, primarily affect these biochemical pathways by poisoning an enzyme or blocking a particular receptor.

The pharmaceutical companies (Big Pharma) spend all of their time, effort, and money on researching drug therapies. Why would Big Pharma rely solely on drug therapies and not only show little interest in natural therapies, but be actively hostile to the idea of using a natural item? The answer to that question involves money.

Natural items, such as Vitamin C and magnesium, are not patentable products. Only unnatural or substances foreign to the body can be patented. Large profits can only be obtained through using a patentable substance. Therefore, the financial incentive for Big Pharma is to obtain and promote the use of patentable substances.

Most pharmaceutical drugs are foreign substances to the body. Being foreign substances, we don't know how these drugs will act in each individual. These drugs have never been in our bodies before we take them. There are no receptors for these foreign substances to bind to and there are no clear detoxifying pathways for our bodies to help excrete these substances. The end result of using drugs is that they usually stay in the body much longer as compared to a natural substances. This prolonged half-life of drugs leads to many of the adverse side effects that plague drug therapies.

I do not mean to imply that drugs do not have their place. They do. If you have pneumonia, antibiotics are invaluable and should be the primary treatment of choice. For an acute heart attack or an acute gastrointestinal bleed, I would want to be in a good emergency room where appropriate life-saving drugs and therapies can be administered. Conventional medicine truly shines in the care of the emergent crises.

However, for the promotion of health and the long-term treatment of chronic illness, I believe that relying solely on a drug therapy will not provide the best outcome. Reliance on the use of drugs that have the ability to poison crucial enzymes and block important receptors will not lead to health. Generally, there will be an increased risk of adverse effects when these drugs are used for a prolonged period of time.

Furthermore, using combinations of different drugs will increase the risk of adverse effects. Frequently, the adverse effects of one drug are generally treated with another drug. An example of this is the use of nonsteroidal anti-inflammatory drugs. Their use causes gastrointestinal problems (see chapter 8). These drug-induced gastrointestinal problems are often treated with antacid drugs which have their own adverse effects (see Chapter 6). Inevitably the use of a multitude of drugs will lead to a downward spiral in one's health.

How common are adverse effects to prescription drugs? Unfortunately, they are very common. A recent study in The Journal of the American Medical Association estimated that there were over 700,000 emergency department visits per year due to adverse drug reactions.[1] Hospitalized patients do not fare any better. It is estimated that there are over 2.2 million adverse drug reactions per year which cause over 106,000 deaths.[2] That is a jumbo-jet full of hospitalized patients dying per day not from their illness but from an adverse drug reaction where the drug was appropriately dispensed.

As a society, we can't continue down the health care path we are on. Drug therapies generally do not treat the underlying cause(s) of an illness and they are too expensive. They also are responsible for a host of adverse effects. We cannot afford to spend the lion's share of health care dollars on therapies that are not promoting health.

This book was written to explain to the reader why some of the most commonly prescribed drugs today may be harmful and why natural therapies should be considered in a treatment program for seven common conditions:

1. Elevated cholesterol levels
2. Depression
3. Diabetes
4. Imbalanced Hormonal System
5. Inflammation
6. Osteoporosis
7. Stomach problems (GERD, ulcers)

These seven conditions were chosen because these are some of the most common problems afflicting patients.

Furthermore, these ailments cost society a great deal of money through the use of expensive drugs that generally do not treat the underlying cause of any illness. If we don't change the way we approach chronic illness, the medical costs will bankrupt our country. In this book, I will give the reader an alternative viewpoint on how to approach the seven common conditions listed above

This book will rely on physiology, biochemistry and common sense. ***Common sense says that the long-term use of items that poison crucial enzymes or block important receptors will not have a positive benefit.*** I wrote this book to provide you with safe and effective natural therapies that treat the underlying cause of your illness. I hope this book helps you to achieve your optimal health.

TO ALL OF OUR HEALTH!

[1] JAMA. 10.18.06. 296(15): 1858-66
[2] JAMA. 4.15.1998. 279:1200-1205

Chapter 2

*Cholesterol-
Lowering Drugs*

INTRODUCTION

Cholesterol-lowering medications have been around for over 30 years. During that time period, more and more medications have become available. Are these drugs working? Do they lower your risk of heart disease? This chapter will help answer these questions.

What is your cholesterol level? It is on the mind of most adults in the United States because Big Pharma has convinced doctors and the public that high cholesterol is ***the cause*** of heart disease. Furthermore, Big Pharma has successfully marketed the message that nearly everyone needs to take drugs to lower their cholesterol levels in order to lower their risk for developing heart disease. This chapter will give you an alternative viewpoint of the cholesterol message. After reading this chapter, you will be able to make an informed decision on whether a cholesterol-lowering medication is the right choice to treat or prevent heart disease.

Cholesterol is the fat-like substance that exists in every cell of the body. In fact, life itself is not possible without adequate amounts of cholesterol in our bodies. This chapter will show you that high cholesterol is <u>NOT</u> the cause of heart disease and, furthermore, that the use of cholesterol-lowering drugs (statins) have never been shown to significantly lower one's risk for developing heart disease. It is this author's opinion that statins should be the last choice (if ever used) for the treatment/prevention of heart disease.

At the turn of the 20th century, infections were the leading cause of death in America as well as the Western world. The discovery and use of antibiotics (after World War II) to treat infections was a major success story of medicine. By the end of the 20th century, heart disease had surpassed infection as the major cause of death.

THE HISTORY OF THE HIGH CHOLESTEROL=HEART DISEASE HYPOTHESIS

After World War II, Ancel Keys, a doctor of physiology, published a paper that reported a link between dietary fat intake and the development of coronary heart disease.[1] He published data comparing the rates of heart disease versus the fat in the diet of six western countries. This information has been made available to every medical student since its publication. From Dr. Keys' analysis, it appeared as if there was a direct relationship between the increased intake of fat in the diet and the increased mortality from heart disease. This study was seized upon as the missing link in treating and overcoming the leading cause of death—heart disease. In fact, this study is still touted as the proof of the cholesterol=heart disease hypothesis.

However, Dr. Keys only included six countries in his now famous work. Dr. Keys had actually studied the relationship between dietary fat and heart disease in 16 other Western countries. When the information from all of the 22 countries studied was analyzed, Dr. Keys' previous assertion of a relationship between dietary fat and heart disease suddenly was not so clear. In fact, upon further analysis of his data, Dr. Keys had 'cherry-picked' the data that supported the link between dietary fat and heart disease. In other words, he only chose those countries that supported his hypothesis. Of course, this was never publicized by the media.

Since that time, Western medicine has been obsessed with the idea that dietary fat and the fat-like substance cholesterol is the cause of heart disease. Furthermore, conventional medicine has claimed that by lowering fat (cholesterol) in the diet or with the use of drug therapies, you can lower the incidence and mortality from heart disease.

Over the last 50 years, we have been inundated with low fat foods, drugs that block fat absorption, drugs that block cholesterol synthesis, food pyramids that promote lowering the fat (cholesterol) in our diets and other measures designed to decrease the cholesterol in our diets and bodies. What do we have to show for all the time and money spent on the cholesterol-lowering idea? What we have is an extremely obese population suffering the ravages of heart disease. In fact, heart disease is still the number one killer. Americans have become the heaviest people on the face of the planet. Chronic illness is rampant. Maybe the advice we have been given over all these years is not correct. In fact, I will make an argument that most of the conventional advice about cholesterol is wrong.

CHOLESTEROL: A TRUE VILLAIN?

If you would believe the media, the AMA, the government, and almost all of the health care agencies, cholesterol is a terrible substance and we need to do whatever we can to lower cholesterol to its lowest possible level. The conventional message further claims that if we don't lower our cholesterol levels we are bound to get heart disease. Is cholesterol a true villain?

The answer is easy: **no**. As previously mentioned, without cholesterol, life itself is not possible. Cholesterol is a necessary ingredient of every cell in the body. The integrity of each cell membrane is dependant on adequate cholesterol production in the body as well as adequate cholesterol intake from the diet.

Cholesterol is a precursor to the production of all of the adrenal hormones (see Figure 1, page 31). As I described in **_The Miracle of Natural Hormones, 3rd Edition_**, a balanced hormonal system is necessary for achieving and maintaining optimal health. It is impossible to overcome many chronic health conditions including autoimmune disorders, fatigue, fibromyalgia, chronic fatigue syndrome, lowered libido, and cancer if the hormonal system is imbalanced. In addition, an imbalanced hormonal system can lead to allergies, asthma, blood sugar problems, inflammation, difficulty healing, and reproductive problems. Table 1 lists many conditions associated with an imbalanced hormonal system. The use of natural, bioidentical hormones along with a holistic treatment program as described in my book has been effective at helping my patients overcome these disorders.

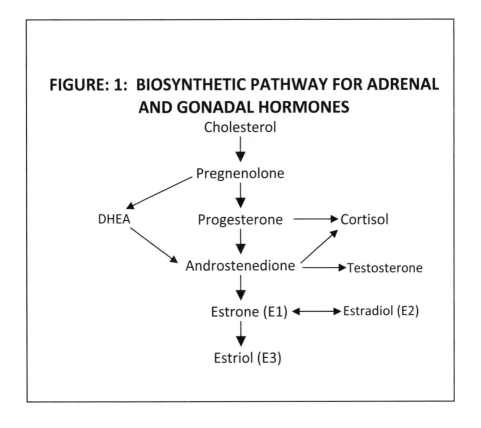

FIGURE: 1: BIOSYNTHETIC PATHWAY FOR ADRENAL AND GONADAL HORMONES

TABLE 1: CONDITIONS ASSOCIATED WITH AN IMBALANCED HORMONAL SYSTEM

Arthritis
Asthma
Autoimmune disorders
Cancer
Chronic fatigue syndrome
Congestive heart failure
Depression
Diabetes
Fatigue
Fibromyalgia
Graves' disease

Hashimoto's disease
Headaches
Heart disease
Hypertension
Hypotension
Hypothyroidism
Immune system diseases
Inflammation
Infertility
Osteoporosis
PMS

HOW ARE THE ADRENAL HORMONES PRODUCED?

Figure 1 (page 31) shows the biosynthetic pathway for the adrenal hormones. The fat-like substance cholesterol is the precursor molecule for <u>all</u> of the adrenal hormones. Adequate cholesterol levels must be maintained to produce optimal amounts of the adrenal hormones. If cholesterol levels are too low, my experience has shown that many times the adrenal hormone production will be suboptimal. Remember, an imbalanced adrenal hormonal system has been associated with a wide range of illnesses—see Table 1.

What happens when the adrenal hormonal system is imbalanced? The production of many (if not all) of the adrenal hormones shown in Figure 1 will decline. The hormonal system can become imbalanced as a result of a variety of circumstances including: a poor diet, vitamin and mineral deficiencies, toxicities, as well as drug therapies which block cholesterol production. My clinical experience has been clear; chronic illness oftentimes goes hand-in-hand with low adrenal hormone production. In fact, I have found it nearly impossible to treat any chronic illness without ensuring an optimally functionally adrenal system.

WHAT IS THE BODY'S RESPONSE TO A DECLINE IN ADRENAL HORMONE PRODUCTION?

In order to achieve your optimal health, an adequate, age-appropriate production of all of the adrenal hormones needs to be maintained. What happens when there is a suboptimal production of the adrenal hormones?

If we look closely at Figure 1, the answer becomes clear: The body will increase the production of cholesterol to try and 'prime' the adrenal pathway. In other words, the body will use cholesterol as a substrate to stimulate the production of the other adrenal hormones. An elevated cholesterol level in this case is the body's normal and expected response to a suboptimal adrenal function.

The last thing you would want to do in this case is to use a drug (such as a statin) to block the production of cholesterol. Our bodies are magnificent. There are many checks and balances to maintain optimal functioning. Statin drugs, by poisoning a crucial enzyme, interfere with the body's normal system of checks and balances. A further discussion of statin drugs can be found later in this chapter.

As previously mentioned, when there is adrenal fatigue with a resultant suboptimal adrenal hormone production, an elevated cholesterol level is the normal and expected response. It is an adaptive response from the body. Instead of killing the messenger (cholesterol) with a statin drug, I believe a better initial approach is to investigate why the adrenal glands are not functioning optimally. In the **_Miracle of Natural Hormones, 3rd_** **_Edition,_** I discuss many of the factors that can result in a hypoadrenal state. Vitamin and mineral imbalances, a poor diet, stress, and thyroid disorders can all cause problems with the adrenal glands. A thorough investigation needs to be undertaken to identify the underlying causes. After identifying the underlying causes, a logical treatment program can be instituted.

My clinical experience has shown that identifying and treating the underlying causes has proven to help many overcome chronic illness and achieve their optimal health. Many times this treatment regimen will include the use of bioidentical hormones along with the appropriate nutritional support.

WHAT HAPPENS WHEN A HYPOADRENAL STATE IS CORRECTED WITH THE USE OF BIOIDENTICAL HORMONES?

As I have described in ***The Miracle of Natural Hormones, 3rd Edition,*** the use of physiologic (low) doses of bioidentical hormones has been very helpful to countless numbers of hypoadrenal patients. Furthermore, when the adrenal hormones are re-balanced, the production of cholesterol will naturally fall—without the use of toxic drugs. No longer will the body have to 'prime' the pump with cholesterol (refer to Figure 1) in order to stimulate adrenal hormone production.

Seventeen years ago a patient came to me with a medical condition that required me to search for a different treatment regimen than what I was taught in medical school. He had a history of a severe coronary artery disease and a very high cholesterol level. This patient was not responding to the commonly used cholesterol-lowering medications. In fact, the drug therapies that he was taking were worsening his condition. I was concerned that he was going to die.

It was the turning point in my medical career when I began to look at the adrenal hormone pathway in more detail.

My father, Ellis, had his first myocardial infarction (MI) or heart attack at age 42 and his first bypass surgery at age 50. Ellis' second bypass occurred at age 58. He had an angioplasty at age 60 and a second angioplasty at 62. All during this time, he had a very high cholesterol level—averaging around 350mg/dl. His cholesterol level was virtually unresponsive to medications. He suffered from a 20-year history of angina, and I never recall him looking or acting well as I was growing up.

When I checked his adrenal hormone levels, I was stunned at the results. Even though he was seeing many good doctors, my father never had his testosterone level checked. When he was 63-years-old, I checked his testosterone level and found it to be extremely low at 1.5 ng/ml (the normal range for men is 3-9 ng/ml). He was also found to be hypothyroid. When I reviewed the medical literature, I was stunned to find a tremendous amount of research that found a direct relationship between hypothyroidism and low testosterone levels both causing heart disease. At this point, I placed him on natural testosterone and Armour® thyroid hormone for his hypothyroid condition. Immediately, my father made a dramatic improvement in his condition. The twenty year angina condition resolved within one week, never to return. Within four weeks, his cholesterol level started falling. I checked his other adrenal hormone levels and treated his hypoadrenal state with a combination of DHEA, progesterone, and pregnenolone. Within six weeks of starting this regimen, his cholesterol level fell to less than 200mg/d—without *the use of a cholesterol-lowering medication.   Most importantly, he never felt or looked better.   After my parents took a trip with their high school friends Donna and Leonard, I received a phone call from Donna.   She asked me what I was prescribing for my father.   When I asked her why, she replied, "David, I haven't seen your father look this good in 30 years.   I want to give Leonard the same thing."*

My father's story is not unique. In fact, I see similar results in many other patients. When an adrenal hormonal imbalance is corrected with physiologic doses of bioidentical, natural hormones, it results in the adrenal glands lowering their production of cholesterol. My father's high cholesterol was not the result of a deficiency of cholesterol-lowering medications. It was the result of an imbalanced adrenal hormonal system. Correcting the hormonal imbalance effectively treated the underlying cause of his high cholesterol condition.

WHAT DOES CHOLESTEROL DO IN THE BODY?

Let's try and answer the question again; is cholesterol a villain? Is it such a bad substance in our bodies that even healthy people need to take medication to dramatically lower cholesterol levels? Absolutely not. In fact, the opposite is true; adequate amounts of cholesterol are necessary for maintaining a healthy immune system and an optimally functioning hormonal system. There are five major functions of cholesterol in the body:

1. CHOLESTEROL AND VITAMIN D

Cholesterol is a precursor to Vitamin D production. Without adequate cholesterol levels, not enough Vitamin D will be produced in the body. Vitamin D is necessary for maintaining a well functioning immune system and strong bones. In addition, Vitamin D deficiency has been linked to a myriad of diseases including cancers of the breast, colon, and prostate. [2 3 4 5 6 7 8 9 10] Vitamin D deficiency is one of the most common nutritional deficiencies that I see in my practice. Optimal Vitamin D levels are nearly impossible to maintain if someone is on a drug that blocks cholesterol production or if there is a very low cholesterol level (<160mg/dl). In fact, the sickest patients I see generally have cholesterol levels below 160mg/dl.

2. CHOLESTEROL IS NECESSSARY FOR FAT AND MINERAL ABSORPTION

Adequate cholesterol levels are necessary for proper absorption and digestion of fats and minerals. Cholesterol is the main ingredient of bile salts, which are stored in the gall bladder. Proper fat digestion is impossible without bile salts. Without bile salts, deficiencies of the fat soluble Vitamins A, D, E, and K will be present. Fat-soluble vitamin deficiencies are common today, due in large part, to cholesterol-lowering drugs.

3. CHOLESTEROL IS INTEGRAL FOR ALL OF THE CELLS OF THE BODY

All of the trillions of cells in our bodies require adequate amounts of cholesterol to form their structures. Cholesterol is the 'glue' that holds the entire lipid cell layers together. It has the ability to give the cell membrane the strength it needs. Without adequate cholesterol production, the cell membranes become leaky. The consequences of leaky cell membranes include the onset of chronic illness and cancer.

4. CHOLESTEROL AND THE NERVOUS SYSTEM

Optimal neurological function is mediated by cholesterol. Cholesterol is necessary for the myelin sheath that covers all of our nerve cells.[11] [12] Cholesterol is important for optimal memory function—it is the primary organic molecule in the brain. Brain fog is very common in those with low cholesterol levels and those on statin drugs. It is also necessary for hormonal production in the brain. Similarly, it is important for neurotransmitter function including serotonin. Low cholesterol levels inhibit serotonin receptors from properly functioning. Cholesterol-lowering drugs have been associated with brain disorders such as neuropathy.[13]

5. CHOLESTEROL AND THE IMMUNE SYSTEM

Cholesterol is necessary for the immune system to fight against infection. Inadequate cholesterol levels in men have been associated with lowered levels and responsiveness of immune system cells. Studies have shown men with lowered cholesterol levels have fewer circulating lymphocytes, total T-cells, and helper T-cells as compared to men with higher cholesterol levels.[14]

Lower cholesterol levels have been associated with a significantly increased risk of being hospitalized for an infectious disease.[15][16] In addition, animal studies have shown that animals have a higher mortality from infections when there are lowered lipids in the blood stream.[17]

HOW IS CHOLESTEROL MADE IN THE BODY?

The liver manufactures cholesterol in the body. Figure 2 details the biosynthetic pathway of cholesterol. As mentioned previously, the liver makes cholesterol for a wide range of functions in the body.

As can be seen from Figure 2, the production of cholesterol is dependent on many different steps. Adequate amounts of

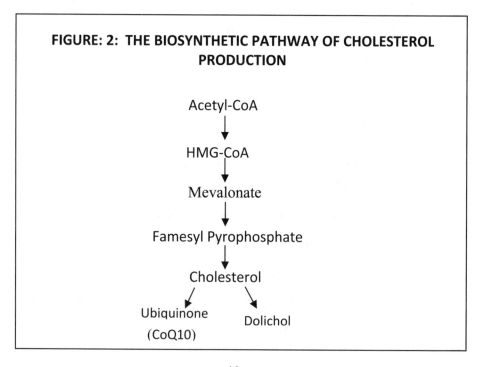

FIGURE: 2: THE BIOSYNTHETIC PATHWAY OF CHOLESTEROL PRODUCTION

Acetyl-CoA

↓

HMG-CoA

↓

Mevalonate

↓

Famesyl Pyrophosphate

↓

Cholesterol

↙   ↘

Ubiquinone   Dolichol
(CoQ10)

vitamins, minerals, and enzymes are necessary to catalyze these reactions. Inadequate levels of any of these agents will inhibit these pathways.

Note that ubiquinone (CoQ10) is produced in the same pathway as cholesterol. Anything that inhibits cholesterol production will invariably inhibit CoQ10 production. A statin drug is an example of a substance that will lower cholesterol levels as well as lower CoQ10 in the body. The consequences of this will be explained later.

DOES LOWERING YOUR CHOLESTEROL PROTECT YOU AGAINST HEART DISEASE?

This is the million dollar question. In the case of Big Pharma, it is a multi-billion dollar question. As mentioned previously, we have been inundated with glossy ads and clever marketing claiming that you will lower your risk for heart disease if you lower your cholesterol levels. Doctors are beseeched by drug representatives with important-looking studies claiming a lowered risk of heart attacks when cholesterol levels are lowered. The ads and research look impressive. However, the Wizard of Oz looked impressive until the curtain was pulled back. Let's look behind the curtain at the research and see what is really true.

THE RESEARCH ON THE RELATIONSHIP BETWEEN LOWERED CHOLESTEROL LEVELS AND THE RISK OF HEART DISEASE

This section will review the research between lowering cholesterol levels and heart disease. The American Heart Association and other mainstream organizations continually stress how important it is to lower your cholesterol. Let's take a closer look at some of the information they provide. The following information is from the American Heart Association web site.[18]

The National Cholesterol Education Program (NCEP) was created in 1985 by the National Heart, Lung, and Blood Institute (NHLBI). The NCEP aims to educate professionals and the public about the benefits of lowering cholesterol levels as a way to reduce the risk for coronary heart disease. The NCEP raises cholesterol awareness through a cooperative effort among groups that include practitioners, public health professionals, community and voluntary organizations (including the American Heart Association), state and local government officials, and healthcare administrators. The media and industry representatives also participate in the program.

The interest groups participating in the NCEP are communicating two important messages to the public and the healthcare professionals who treat them. The first is, "Know your blood cholesterol level. If it's high, you can reduce your risk of heart disease by lowering it."

Patterned after the National High Blood Pressure Education Program, the NCEP is founded on two principles. First, its educational initiatives and messages are based on firm scientific evidence. Second, various public and private healthcare organizations are partners with the NHLBI in developing and carrying out the campaign.

The Adult Treatment Panel III (ATP III) of the NCEP issued an evidence-based set of guidelines on cholesterol management in 2001. Since then, five major clinical trials of statin therapy have been published. A 2004 publication appearing in the journal <u>Circulation</u> reviews the results of these recent trials and assesses their implications for cholesterol management.

Let's look at what is said in the AHA web release. "Know your blood cholesterol level. If it's high, you can reduce your risk of heart disease by lowering it." This is the mantra promoted by conventional medicine—reduced cholesterol levels=reduced heart disease risk. Further along the press release, they cite that this is an 'evidence-based set of guidelines' and they state that five major clinical trials have been published since 2001 supporting their hypothesis.

If reducing cholesterol levels lowers the risk of heart disease, you would assume that people who lower their cholesterol levels will live longer as compared to those who do not lower their cholesterol levels. I believe the most important statistic of any study is the mortality rate—who is alive at the end of the study. Let us take a close look at the mortality rate of those five studies cited by the American Heart Association.

1. ***Heart Protection Study (2002).*** 20,536 adults in the U.K. (aged 40-80) who were at a high risk for heart disease

43

were followed for five years. Patients were randomized into two groups: a placebo group and a group that received Zocor® (simvastatin) 40mg/day. The placebo group had an 85.4% chance of surviving after five years as compared to 87.1% in the Zocor treated group. Therefore, the numbers show an absolute reduction in mortality of 1.7%. Not a huge decline. Dr. Uffe Ravnskov wrote, "Low cholesterol concentrations have been related to depression, cognitive impairment, and suppression of the immune system. Does a reduction of 1.7% in mortality balance these risks?"[19]

2.   Prosper (2002). 5804 adults were examined to look at the effect of Pravachol® (pravastatin) versus placebo in the risk of developing heart disease and stroke. At the end of the trial (three years), the placebo group had 89.5% alive compared to the treatment group of 89.7% alive. A 0.2% difference. Again, not a huge difference. One notable side effect was that cancer was significantly increased in the treatment group.

3.   ALLHAT (2003). 10,355 adults over 55 years old were randomized to receive either Pravachol or usual care. The mortality results show that at the end of the study (six years) there were 84.7% of the control group alive and

85.1% of the Pravachol-treated group alive—a 0.4% difference. Again, not much of a difference.

4. ASCOT-LLA. 19,342 hypertensive patients, 40 to 79 years old having risk factors for cardiovascular disease were randomized into one of two groups; one group took a placebo and one group took Lipitor®. Lipitor® did reduce the number of cardiac events compared to the placebo, but did not significantly change the overall mortality. At the end of the 3.3 year study, 95.9% of the control group was alive versus 96.4% of the Lipitor®-treated group. A 0.5% difference—a miniscule difference.

5. PROVE-IT. 4,162 patients who had a heart attack or angina were randomized to either taking Lipitor® or Pravachol®. The results showed an absolute reduction in the death rate of Lipitor® was 2.2% versus 3.2% from Pravachol®. There was no control group.

So, these are the five studies the NCEP has cited which 'prove' that lowering your cholesterol will lead to lowering your risk of heart disease. None of these studies showed a dramatic decrease in the mortality of those who took a drug to lower their cholesterol levels. In four of the above studies, there was a slight decline (average of 0.775%) in mortality in the treated group versus the placebo group. However, when the risks of the statins (which are covered in the next section) are considered, I believe it

45

will be clear that using a drug to block cholesterol function clearly has more risks than benefits. There are much safer ways to lower your risk of developing heart disease than taking a statin drug.

There are many more studies that refute the 'lower cholesterol=lower risk of heart disease' hypothesis. It is beyond this book to review them all. I refer the reader to three wonderful books for more information:

1. *Malignant Medical Myths* by Joel Kauffman
2. *The Cholesterol Myths,* by Uffe Ravnskov
3. *Hidden Truth about Cholesterol-Lowering Drugs* by Shane Ellison

WHAT ARE THE RISKS OF LOWERING CHOLESTEROL LEVELS? A HIGHER DEATH RATE

There are many risks associated with lowering cholesterol levels. The elderly are particularly sensitive to lowered cholesterol levels. In fact, one study showed that in the elderly female, a lower cholesterol level (<155mg/dl) was associated with a 5.2 times higher death rate as compared to a woman with a cholesterol level of 272mg/dl.[20] Other studies have also shown that in women of all ages and men over 55, high cholesterol may actually result in a decreased mortality.[21] A study in Austria which included over 150,000 subjects, showed that low cholesterol levels predict premature death in men of all ages and in women over the age of 50.[22]

My clinical experience has been clear: when total cholesterol levels markedly decrease, death is imminent. The Framingham study showed that the odds of cancer death were two-fold higher if a large fall in total cholesterol occurred over any four year period.[23] More about the relationship with longevity and cholesterol levels will be discussed later in this chapter. Any rapid decline in cholesterol levels needs a full investigation to determine the reasons why it has fallen.

CHOLESTEROL-LOWERING DRUGS: POISONING A CRUCIAL ENZYME

It is impossible to disrupt a normal biochemical pathway for the long term and expect a good clinical result to occur. *In other words, you can't poison a crucial enzyme for the long-term and expect a good result.*

Statin drugs poison the enzyme HMG-CoA Reductase, which is a precursor enzyme to cholesterol production (see Figure 1). Examples of statin drugs include Lipitor®, Crestor®, Mevacor®, Pravachol®, and Zocor®. When you understand the biosynthetic pathway for cholesterol production (see Figure 2), it doesn't make physiological sense and it certainly doesn't make common sense to poison a crucial enzyme necessary for the production of cholesterol. If what I say is true, then why are statin drugs still prescribed?

Follow the money. The top two drugs that bring in the

most money for Big Pharma are statins. In 2004, Lipitor® was the most prescribed drug in the United States. Over seven million prescriptions for Lipitor® were written, bringing in revenue of over 7.7 billion dollars. The next most profitable drug was Zocor® which brought in over 4.5 billion dollars of revenue.[24] Statin drugs are one of the most profitable class of medications for Big Pharma.

WHAT DO STATINS DO IN THE BODY?

Statins are a class of medications that poison an enzyme, HMG-CoA Reductase. Figure 3 shows where statins interact in the biosynthetic pathway for cholesterol metabolism. By poisoning the HMG-CoA Reductase enzyme, Acetyl CoA cannot be converted into HMG-CoA. Therefore, all of the substances 'downstream' from HMG-CoA will also be reduced.

If you look at Figure 3 (page 49), you can see the consequences of taking a statin drug. Statin drugs do what they advertise; they lower cholesterol levels. However, they also result in lowered levels of CoQ10. Lowered levels of CoQ10 can result in muscle weakness, congestive heart failure as well as other problems. More about CoQ10 will be found later in this chapter.

DO STATINS LOWER CHOLESTEROL LEVELS?

Absolutely. They work as advertised. By poisoning the HMG-CoA Reductase enzyme, cholesterol levels will be reduced.

As I explained previously, be careful what you wish for; a lowered cholesterol level may not be the most desired result, particularly as you get older.

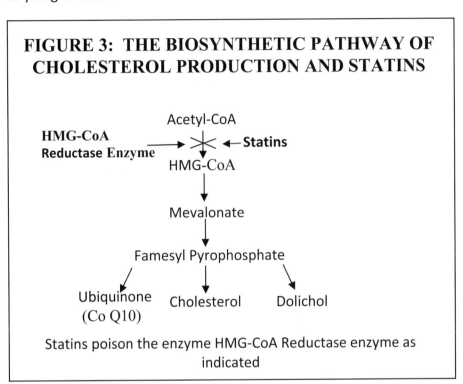

FIGURE 3: THE BIOSYNTHETIC PATHWAY OF CHOLESTEROL PRODUCTION AND STATINS

Statins poison the enzyme HMG-CoA Reductase enzyme as indicated

DO STATINS HAVE SIDE EFFECTS?

Yes. A lot of them. When any crucial biochemical pathway (see Figure 3), is poisoned, adverse effects are bound to occur. What are the adverse effects of statins?

1. Muscle pain and weakness. This is the most common side effect reported. Published data reports that this side effect occurs 1-5% the time. However, I believe the numbers are much higher. At the American College of Physicians annual meeting

(2006), one doctor claimed that, "I believe the number is much higher. In my practice, it's probably 20%, at least."[25] Why would this occur? If you look at Figure 2, it becomes clear. The depletion of CoQ10 would lead one to assume that muscle aches and weakness will occur.

CoQ10 is a biocatalyst that facilitates the activities of enzymes. It is necessary for maintaining optimal muscle function. CoQ10 is essential for cellular energy production. The heart muscle contains one of the largest amounts of CoQ10 in the body.

If statin-induced muscle pain and weakness progresses, it can lead to a potentially fatal condition called rhabdomyolysis. Doctors will frequently monitor their patients on statin drugs for an elevated muscle enzyme called creatine kinase (CK). When CK levels elevate, it suggests a serious problem with the statin drug. However, you can get serious problems with statin drugs even without elevated CK levels.

How do you avoid rhabdomyolosis and other muscle problems with statins? Keep your CoQ10 levels elevated. If you take a statin drug, you should be prescribed CoQ10 to take with that statin. RECOMMENDATION: I suggest taking 150-300mg of CoQ10/day if you are taking a statin.

2. Body aches and pains. Complaints of body aches and pains are common with statin users. It may be related to CoQ10 depletion described above. There have been many case reports of patients complaining of body aches and pains with the onset of taking a statin. These symptoms often resolve after discontinuing the statin.

3. Heart Failure. Today, congestive heart failure is occurring at an epidemic rate in the U.S. Each year approximately 550,000 new cases are diagnosed. Heart failure affects 1% of people aged 50 years, 5% of those aged 75 years and older and 25% of those over 85 years. Approximately 50% of those with heart failure will die within five years of their diagnosis. Heart failure is the most common reason Medicare patients are admitted to the hospital.[26]

What could be fueling this epidemic of heart failure? Statin use is certainly one cause. Researchers at the East Texas Medical Center studied 20 patients with normal cardiac function. After six months of Lipitor®, 66% developed problems in diastole—the filling phase of the heart cycle. This is the same problem many congestive heart failure patients have. The researchers' explanation for their findings were, "Statins can cause a dose-related depletion in an essential nutrient known as Coenzyme Q10. ...The heart is especially susceptible because it uses so much energy."[27] There have been at least nine controlled studies on the treatment of heart disease with CoQ10. All nine studies have shown the effectiveness of CoQ10. Over 300 international papers on CoQ10 use in heart disease have had the same conclusion: CoQ10 improves heart muscle function.[28]

As previously mentioned, statins inhibit CoQ10 production. The heart is the body's largest muscle and contains the largest concentration of the body's CoQ10. Statin use results in a depletion of the stores of CoQ10 both in the body and in the heart. This depletion will lead to myopathy (muscle aches and pains) throughout the body and may eventually lead to congestive heart failure. As previously stated, supplementing with CoQ10 would be the prudent course if you are going to take a statin.

4. Brain fog and dementia. Adequate cholesterol levels are necessary for proper brain function. Much of the brain is composed of fats (the majority of which is cholesterol). Over 50% of dry weight of the cerebral cortex (thinking part of the brain) is cholesterol.[29] The elderly are particularly sensitive to decreases in cholesterol levels. Cholesterol is the repair item for both the brain and the body; when there is damage to body tissue, cholesterol is produced locally in large amounts to help heal the area. My clinical experience has been clear: Those with the lowest cholesterol levels (<150mg/dl) consistently exhibit more brain fog and dementia as compared to those with higher cholesterol levels.

5. Cancer. All of the cholesterol drugs, including the older medications, the fibrates (clofibrate and gemfibrozol) and the newer statins have been associated with an increased rate of cancer.[30] In rodents, statins have been shown to cause cancer in multiple studies.[31] Breast cancer rates in humans that took statins were shown to increase by 1,200% (relative risk).[32] The connection between statins and cancer is hard to pin down since most of the studies do not last for long periods of time. When you look at the mechanism of action of the statins, and the resultant depletion of cholesterol and CoQ10, I believe long-term statin use will inevitably lead to a significantly increased risk of cancer.

6. Depression. There is a long list of medical articles showing the connection between depression and low cholesterol levels. Cholesterol, being the precursor for the adrenal hormones, must be produced in adequate amounts in order to help maintain hormonal balance in the body. When the adrenal hormones become imbalanced, one of the key problems that can develop is depression. By lowering cholesterol, statins can not only cause depression, they also have a tendency to exacerbate a depressive condition.

DO STATINS PREVENT HEART ATTACKS?

As mentioned in the previous studies, statins have a slight benefit in preventing a heart attack. However, this benefit is probably not from the ability of statins to reduce cholesterol levels. Statins have been found to have an anti-inflammatory effect. It is probably this anti-inflammatory effect or some other mechanism that helps statins slightly lower the risk for heart attack (approximately 1%). However, the adverse effects of statins explained above certainly outweigh any small percentage benefit. Furthermore, there are much safer and effective ways to lower your risk of heart attack such as weight loss, lowering homocysteine levels with B Vitamins, smoking cessation, taking Vitamin C and fish oils, etc.

DOES LOWERING YOUR CHOLESTEROL INCREASE YOUR LONGEVITY?

If it is true (as Big Pharma claims) that statins significantly lower your risk for heart disease, then you would expect that studies would show that having a lowered cholesterol will result in a longer life-span.

The Journal of the American Medical Association reported on a study of 5,170 subjects taking Pravachol® versus 5,185 subjects treated with 'usual care' (changes in lifestyle).[33] Pravachol® was found to be more effective at reducing cholesterol (17% versus 8%) and 'bad' LDL cholesterol (28% versus 11%). The study lasted four years. The reduction in cholesterol levels made headlines, but the all-cause mortality findings did not. The all-cause mortality is a measure of the number of people who died from any cause during the study. The all-cause mortality between the two groups was nearly equal. The coronary heart disease rates were not different between the control group and the Pravachol® group.

The Framingham study is one of the longest ongoing research projects studying heart disease. In 1987, researchers reported that after 30 years of follow up, there is no increased overall mortality with subjects with high cholesterol for those over 50 years of age. Furthermore, researchers reported that falling cholesterol levels were found to increase the cardiovascular death rate—a 14% increase for every 1mg/dl drop in cholesterol levels.[34]

A study of 11,563 subjects found that subjects with cholesterol levels below 160mg/dl had a 49% increase in all-cause mortality as compared to those subjects with a cholesterol level over 160mg/dl. Non-cardiac deaths increased by 2.27 times in the low cholesterol group as compared to the control group. The most frequent cause of non-cardiac death was cancer.[35] Other studies have also found a correlation with low cholesterol levels and increased risk for mortality from cancer of the lung, liver, pancreas and bone marrow as well as an increased risk of death from respiratory, hepatic and digestive disease.[36] Another study of 5,491 men aged 45 to 68 years of age found that falling cholesterol levels—from 180-239mg/dl to <180mg/dl—were associated with a 30% higher risk of all-cause mortality and a significantly increased risk of death from cancers of the esophagus, prostate, and bone marrow.[37]

In 997 elderly patients (>70 years old) studied, researchers found no correlation between elevated cholesterol levels and increases in mortality from coronary heart disease, all-cause mortality, or hospitalization from heart attacks or angina.[38] There are many other studies that indicate that lowering your cholesterol level will not prolong your life.

Cholesterol is a vital substance for every cell in the body. *It is deleterious to poison a crucial enzyme for the long-term and expect a good result.*

SHOULD ANYONE TAKE A STATIN?

Unless you have an extremely rare condition called hereditary hypercholesteremia, whereby the cholesterol and triglyceride levels may approach the thousands, I don't feel you need to take a drug that poisons a crucial biosynthetic pathway. Even for those with hereditary hypercholesteremia, there is little research showing a long-term benefit from statin use. When you use a drug for the long-term that poisons a crucial biosynthetic pathway, you are asking for trouble.

The benefits from using statin drugs have been overstated. Dr. Joel Kaufman, author of *Malignant Medical Myths* (highly recommended) summed it up by writing, "The benefits of the statin drugs in reducing mortality are exaggerated being only about 0.3% per year from the most favorable trials. This is not as great as the omega-3 supplements. The tendency of drug makers to make public the results of only the most favorable trials indicates that even the minor benefits described...might be exaggerated. Statins are the drug class most likely to bankrupt Medicare, Medicaid, and other insurance plans without any significant benefits."[39]

NATURAL THERAPIES TO LOWER CHOLESTEROL LEVELS: NIACIN AND FISH OIL

Niacin is found in red meat, chicken, turkey, beans, and grains. Niacin (Vitamin B3) may be the most perfect item in treating coronary artery disease. It is less expensive and more effective at improving cholesterol numbers and much safer than any statin drug. Niacin has been shown to decrease LDL-cholesterol and triglycerides as well as increase HDL-cholesterol. It also decreases lipoprotein(a) which is a risk factor for heart disease. Niacin has also been shown to reduce the incidence of recurrent, nonfatal heart attacks risk by 27% and the number of strokes by 26%.[40]

HOW TO DOSE NIACIN: Niacin can be taken as an immediate release, extended release, slow release, or no flush supplement. I recommend the immediate or extended release supplement. However, I do not recommend taking slow release niacin as there have been reports of liver toxicity with this form. Also, I do not recommend taking 'no-flush' niacin as it does not provide the cardiovascular benefits listed above. The main side effect with taking niacin is a flushing reaction. I recommend you take niacin once or twice per day. Niacin doses need to be individualized. Doses can range from 500mg to 5,000mg/day. The larger doses (over 500mg/day) should be taken only with physician supervision.

Fish oil has been shown to lower elevated triglyceride levels as well as prevent blood clots and slow plaque growth. It helps prevent sudden cardiac death and can normalize heart arrhythmias. Not bad for an inexpensive supplement. HOW TO DOSE FISH OIL: Fish oil doses range from 1,200 to 3,000mg per day.

FINAL THOUGHTS

Statin drugs have been touted as the miracle cure for heart disease, inflammation, cancer, osteoporosis, and other illnesses. The media campaign promoting the use of statins is impressive.

However, I would advise the reader to do their own research and make their own conclusions. The benefits of the statin drugs are overstated by Big Pharma. Just as Big Pharma overstated the benefits of conventional hormone replacement therapy (with synthetic hormones) for over 25 years, the same event is presently occurring with the statins.

Research has shown that higher cholesterol levels are protective for women and men over the age of 55. Cholesterol is not a substance to be feared; we cannot live without adequate amounts of cholesterol.

It all comes down to physiology and biochemistry. Science does not lie. I do not feel it is in the best interest of most patients, for the long term, to poison a crucial enzyme such as HMG-CoA reductase. Dr. Uffe Ravnskof, author of the excellent book, **_Cholesterol Myths_** sums up why you should avoid long-term statin use by stating, "It is simply stupidity to think that you can poison important metabolic enzymes for decades without serious consequences."[41]

---

[1] Keys, A. Atherosclerosis: A problem in the new public health Journal of Mt. Sinai Hospital. 20, 118-139, 1953

[2] In. J. Epidem. 1980 Sep;9(3):227-31

[3] Lancet. 1985 Feb. 9;1(8424):307-9

[4] J. Natl. Cancer Inst. 1996. Oct 2;88(19) 1375-82

[5] Lancet. 1989. Jan. 28;1(8631):188-91

[6] Braz. J. Med. Biol. Res. 2002. Jan;35(1):1-9

[7] Prev. Med. 1990. Nov;19)6):614-22

[8] Int. J. Epidem. 1990. Dec;19(4):820-4

[9] Anticancer Res. 1990. Sept-Oct.;10(5a): 1307-11

[10] Cancer Causes Control. 1998. Aug;9(4):425-32

[11] Simons, M. Assembly of myelin by association of proteolipid protein with cholesterol- and galactosylceramide-rich membrane domains. J. of Cell. Biology. 2000. Oct. 2;151(1):1143-54.

[12] Arteriolsclerosis. Throm. Vasc. Biol. 2004;24:806-15

[13] Smith, D.F. Southern Med. J. 96(12):1265-1267, Dec. 2003.

[14] Muldoon, M.F. Immune systems differences in men with hypo- or hypercholesterolemia. Clin. Immunol. Immunopathol. 1997;84:145-9

[15] Iribarren, C. Serum total cholesterol and risk of hospitalization , and death from respiratory disease. Intern. J. of Epidem. 26. 1191-1202. 1997

[16] Iribarren, C. Cohort study of serum total cholesterol and in-hospital incidence of infectious disease. Epidem. and Infection. 121. 335-47. 1998

[17] Netera, M.G. Low-density lipoprotein receptor-deficient mice are protected against lethal endotoxemia and server Gram-negative infections. J. Clin. Invest. 1996;97:1366-72

[18] Accessed from: www.americanheart.org/presenter.jhtml?identifier=4638. Accessed 4.2.06

[19] Ravnskov, U. BMJ. 2002;324:789

[20] Forette, B. Cholesterol as a risk factor for mortality in elderly women. Lancet. 1:868-870. 1989

[21] Ravnskov, U. High cholesterol may protect against infections an atherosclerosis. Q. J. Med. 2003;96:927-34

[22] Ulmer, H. Why Eve is not Adam: prospective follow-up in 149650 women and men of cholesterol and othe risk factors related to cardiovascular and all-cause mortality. J. of Womens Health. Jan-Feb;13(1):41-53.

[23] Sharp, SF. Time trends in serum cholesterol before cancer death. Epidemiology 8:132-6. 1997

[24] Pharmacytimes.com/article.cfm?ID=2534

[25] Quote from Dr. Douglas Paauw as reported in `FP News. July 1, 2006. p. 16.

[26] American Heart Association. Heart Disease and Stroke Facts, 2004, Dallas: AHA, 2004.

[27] From www.smartmoney.com. November, 2003.

[28] Langsjoen, P. Introduction to Coenzyme Q10. From: http://faculty.washinton.edu/~ely/coenzq10.html

[29] Fallon, S. The Dangers of Statin Drugs: What you haven't been told about cholesterol-lowering medication. From: www. Mercola.com

[30] Newman, T. Carcinogenicity of lipid-lowering drugs. JAMA. 1.3.1996. Vol. 275, No. 1

[31] Newman, TB. JAMA. 1996;2755-60

[32] Sacks, FM. N. Eng. J. Med. 1996;385;1001-9

[33] JAMA. Dec. 18, 2002. 18;288:2998-3007

[34] Anderson, K. Cholesterol and mortality. 30 years of follow-up from the Framingham study. JAMA. Vol. 257. No. 16, 4.24.1987

[35] Behar, S. Low total cholesterol is associated with high total mortality in patients with coronary heart disease. Eur. Heart Journal. 1997. 18, 52-59

[36] Neaton, J. Serum cholesterol level and mortality findings for men screened in the multiple risk factor intervention trial. Arch. Intern. Med. 192;152. 1490=1500

[37] Iribarren, C. Low serum cholesterol and mortality. Which is the cause and which is the effect. Circulation. 1995;92:2396-2403

[38] Krumholz, H. Lack of association between cholesterol and coronary heart disease mortality and morbidity and all-cause mortality in persons older than 70 years. JAMA. Vol. 272. No. 17. November 2, 1994.

[39] Kauffman, J. Malignant Medical Myths. Infinity Pub. 2006.

[40] J. Am. Cardiology. 1986 Dec;8(6):1245-55

[41] http://www.healthmyths.net/uffe.html. Accessed: 10.28.06

Chapter 3

New Studies on Cholesterol-Lowering Drugs

INTRODUCTION

It has been nearly two years since I wrote the first edition of ***Drugs That Don't Work and Natural Therapies That Do.*** During this time, the idea that lowering cholesterol with medications in order to prevent/treat heart disease has gained even more momentum in the media. Numerous studies have been released, some with positive headlines, some with negative headlines, about the use of cholesterol-lowering medications. This chapter was written to update you on the new studies and to show you how to read between the media headlines to get the real truth behind cholesterol-lowering medications.

Perhaps the study that has made the biggest media splash was the JUPITOR study. The Wall Street Journal headline shouted, "Cholesterol Drug Cuts Heart Risk in Healthy Patients".[1] The article went on to claim that the statin drug, "...Crestor sharply lowered {the} risk of heart attacks among apparently healthy patients in a major study...". It was reported that Crestor "reduced the risk of heart-related death, heart attacks, and other serious cardiac problems by 44% compared with those given a placebo."[2]

When I saw the headlines and the advertising on television, I began to wonder, "Was I wrong? Do I have to rethink my position on statin drugs?" I decided the best course of action was to go to the original article, dissect it, and then determine whether my previous assumptions about cholesterol-lowering medications were still valid.   Let's go through this article together.

THE JUPITOR STUDY

The Jupitor study looked at 17,802 apparently healthy men and women with low density lipoprotein (LDL) cholesterol levels of less than 130mg/dl and a high sensitivity C-reactive protein level (CRP--a marker of inflammation) of 2.0mg/L or higher. The subjects were randomized to taking 20mg/day of Crestor or placebo. Then they were followed for the occurrence of a heart attack, stroke, hospitalization for unstable angina, or death from cardiovascular disease.   The study was supposed to run for five years but was stopped at 1.9 years because of the positive results.

The article in the Wall Street Journal and other newspapers glowingly reported that Crestor reduced the risk of heart-related death, heart attacks, and other serous cardiac problems by 44% compared to those given a placebo. In fact the

Wall Street Journal article described Crestor as "poised for orbit". Heart disease is our number one killer and it has been our number one killer for many years. Any substance that can reduce the risk of death by 44% can change the face of medicine.

A CLOSER LOOK AT THE DATA

When I analyzed the original article, I saw a much different picture than what the media headlines were proclaiming. The first item I look at with any research article is who is funding the research. This study was funded by Big Pharma Astra Zeneca, the producers and marketers of Crestor. Furthermore, the lead author holds the patent on the CRP test and this patent had been licensed to Astra Zeneca. If the media headlines were true, then the market share of Crestor and the CRP test would increase exponentially. The rest of the disclosure listed all the Big Pharma companies who each of the authors were affiliated with. Once I saw the relationships between the authors and Big Pharma, I knew to take a very close look at the rest of the article. Here is what I found.

This study was reported to be composed of "healthy" individuals, free of heart disease. However, one of the prime screening criteria was to only have individuals with an elevated CRP level. CRP is a marker for inflammation. Having an elevated CRP level should cause a doctor to search for causes of inflammation. I do not think a healthy person should have an elevated CRP level. What can cause an elevated CRP level? Any condition that promotes inflammation can cause an elevated CRP. This can include diabetes, autoimmune disorders and heart disease.

DID THE DEATH RATE TRULY DECLINE BY 44%?

One of the main claims by the media was that the death rate significantly declined in "healthy" people who took Crestor for 1.9 years (the length of the study). The actual figures for the total number of people who died during the study were 198 (out of 8901—2.2%) in the Crestor arm and 247 (out of 8901—2.7%) in the placebo arm.

Is the change in the number of deaths between the treated group and the control group important? Well, it depends on what you consider important. If you use the less accurate relative risk, these numbers say that Crestor will result in a 20% relative risk decline in death from any cause (2.2%/2.7%). However, the relative risk should not be used to make clinical decisions. Clinical decisions are better made with the more accurate absolute risk value.

The New England Journal of Medicine states, "Absolute differences in risk are more clinically important than relative reductions in risk in deciding whether to recommend drug therapy."[3] In this study, the absolute risk for death due to any cause was 0.5%. According to this study, this means that you would have to treat 200 patients for 1.9 years with Crestor in order to prevent one death. The cost of 200 patients taking Crestor for 1.9 years is $302,000. Now, you can begin to see why Big Pharma would report these numbers in this misleading way; the dollars are staggering.

Once I saw these numbers, I knew I was not wrong. Unfortunately, you cannot rely on media headlines. It is important to read between the headlines and go to the original source. So, should we all take Crestor for the rest of our lives? Hogwash. I say, for those with an elevated CRP test—a better course is to search for why the CRP is elevated and treat it. What lowers CRP? Cleaning up the diet, eliminating refined foods, drinking adequate amounts of water, treating thyroid problems, and taking vitamin C are all effective at lowering CRP levels. These ideas are less expensive, do not promote adverse effects, and are a good long-term strategy to helping the body avoid chronic illness such as heart disease.

CONGESTIVE HEART FAILURE AND CHOLESTEROL LEVELS

Congestive heart failure is rising at epidemic rates. Between 1980 and 2006, hospitalizations for heart failure have increased by 230%.[4] This is not due to the aging population. Something is causing this dramatic increase. I believe it is due to the overuse of statin drugs.

In December, 2008, researchers released a study looking at 17,791 hospitalized heart failure patients admitted to various hospitals across the United States.[5] The authors were looking at the correlation between in-hospital mortality and the total cholesterol levels.

What the researchers found was astounding. The higher the cholesterol levels were, the lower the death rate. Conversely, the lower the cholesterol levels were, the higher the death rate. The numbers are shown in the table below.

Total Cholesterol(mg/dl)	<118	119-145	146-179	>180
Mean Total Cholesterol	98	131	158	213
Statin Use (%)	58	50	43	34
Died in Hospital (%)	3.3	2.5	2.0	1.3

All of the numbers shown in Table 1 above reached statistical significance. So, what can you take from the above information in the chart? In those with congestive heart failure, lower cholesterol levels are associated with more deaths. Furthermore, you can see that statin drug use was associated with more deaths in those studied.

The authors concluded that,"Low cholesterol levels are associated with poor prognosis in patients hospitalized with heart failure." I would like to know why this study did not make media headlines.

ENHANCE STUDY: VYTORIN

Vytorin was heavily promoted by Big Pharma to prevent cardiovascular disease. Vytorin is a combination drug consisting of the statin medication Zocor and the drug Zetia, which inhibits cholesterol absorption from the gut. Vytorin sales peaked in 2007 with over $5 billion in sales.

The ENHANCE trial was designed to look at the effect of Zocor versus Vytorin (i.e., Zocor and Zetia) in patients with familial hypercholesterolemia. Specifically, the authors were looking to see if the cholesterol-lowering therapies resulted in less thickening of the artery walls, which is a sign of atherosclerosis.

The results showed that cholesterol levels, LDL-cholesterol levels, triglyceride levels, and C-reactive protein levels all declined significantly in both groups, but to a greater extent in the Vytorin group as compared to the Zocor group.

However, the change in the thickness of the artery walls failed to decline in either group and actually increased in the those taking Vytorin. How can you reconcile this?

Well, if you believe the cholesterol=heart disease hypothesis, you can't reconcile this study. I believe this study is one more nail-in-the-coffin of the cholesterol=heart disease hypothesis.

A couple of observations on the ENHANCE study. First, the adverse effects in the Zocor group were reported to be 30% and in the Vytorin group were at 34%. A drug should have a big upside to it if has an adverse effect rate of 30%. No upside was reported in this study. Finally, Big Pharma delayed the reporting of the ENHANCE trial in order to maximize profits. Once the results of the failed trial were announced, market share for the drug began to decline. Although the lipid parameters (total cholesterol, LDL-cholesterol, etc.,) declined, there was no corresponding decline in the thickness of the arteries. In fact the opposite occurred; the thickness of the arteries increased as cholesterol levels fell the most. Certainly this study gives little reason to take either a statin drug or Vytorin.

FINAL THOUGHTS

Recent studies continue to point out problems with the statin drugs. In the U.S., we take more statin drugs than any other people on the face of the earth. Yet we do not see the benefits of these drugs. In fact, we are starting to see problems with the statins, such as the epidemic rise of congestive heart failure.

The main problem with lipid-lowering drugs is that they do not result in a reversal of cardiac disease nor are they a cost effective way to prevent cardiac disease. Cardiac disease is not caused by a lack of a lipid-lowering drug. It is a result of nutritional and hormonal imbalances. Only by correcting the underlying cause of heart disease will we begin to see a real decline in the illness.

[1] Wall Street Journal. Novemnber 10, 2008
[2] Wall Street Journal. Novemnber 10, 2008
[3] NEJM.Vol. 359:2280-2282. Nov. 20, 2008
[4] FP News. 12.16.08
[5] Americn Heart Journal. Vol. 156. N.6. Dec. 2008

Chapter 4

Diabetic Medications

INTRODUCTION

I have been interested in helping patients with diabetes for over 30 years. My father developed type 2 diabetes during my childhood. Over the next 20 years, I watched him suffer from the ravages of type 2 diabetes, which spurred me to find safe and effective methods to help diabetic patients overcome their illness and live normal lives.

In the vast majority of people, type 2 diabetes, which affects over 90% of patients diagnosed with diabetes, can be effectively managed with appropriate diet, lifestyle changes, and nutrient supplementation. None of the commonly used prescription medications have been shown to alter the course of the illness. This chapter will provide you with the information necessary to help you avoid, as well as overcome diabetes.

Diabetes is a group of illnesses which share a common biomarker--elevated blood glucose levels. Diabetes is diagnosed when the fasting blood sugar is greater than 125mg/dl.

Prediabetes is defined by a fasting blood sugar between 100-124mg/dl. Normal fasting blood sugar should be less than 100mg/dl. Diabetes is a disease in which the body does not produce enough insulin or is unable to properly utilize insulin to control blood sugar. According to the American Diabetes Association, in the United States there are 23.6 million children and adults, approximately 8% of the population, who have diabetes.[1] Another 57 million Americans have prediabetes. Unbelievably, over 40% of the U.S. adult population has diabetes or prediabetes.[2][3] The economic costs of diabetes are staggering; in 2007, the total estimated cost of diabetes was $174 billion, which includes $58 billion in reduced national productivity.[4] Diabetes is the fifth deadliest disease in the U.S.[5] It is estimated that diabetes contributes to over 233,000 deaths per year. Diabetes is associated with a host of serious illnesses including: blindness, cataracts, depression, heart disease and stroke, high blood pressure, kidney disease, nervous system damage and amputations.

Diabetes is a terrible illness. Anyone who watches a loved one go through the downward spiral of diabetes understands this. I will show you that the most commonly prescribed drugs, the type 2 oral diabetic medications, do little to reverse the course of this illness. In fact, most of these drugs have severe adverse effects and should not be used at all. For the vast majority of diabetics (type 2), oral drugs are not needed. Lifestyle changes should be the treatment of choice. There will be more about this later.

WHAT HAPPENS IN DIABETES?

We eat food to provide the body with the raw materials to maintain health and produce energy. After we eat food, the digestion process breaks food down to glucose. This causes blood sugar to rise. The islet cells (beta cells) of the pancreas respond to this rise in glucose by producing the hormone insulin. Insulin's role is to facilitate the entry of glucose into the cells in order to produce energy. Diabetics either produce too little insulin or cannot effectively utilize the insulin they are producing. The end result in diabetes is the elevation of blood sugar.

PROBLEMS WITH ELEVATED BLOOD SUGAR

The body is not designed to tolerate elevated blood sugar. The kidneys try to eliminate the excess sugar by producing large amounts of urine. The excess sugar that cannot be eliminated by the kidneys can cause an adverse chemical reaction in the cells of the body which is known as glycation. Glycation is a chemical reaction with a sugar molecule and a protein that impairs the normal functioning of the cells of the body by producing advanced glycation endproducts (AGE's). These AGE's are implicated in the most common chronic illnesses including diabetes, cardiovascular diseases, Alzheimer's disease, cancer, peripheral neuropathy, and blindness (from diabetes). AGE's are eliminated from the body very slowly. Avoiding diabetes and elevated blood sugars significantly reduces the levels of AGE's produced in the body.

TYPE 1 AND TYPE 2 DIABETES

There are two major classifications of diabetes known as type 1 and type 2 diabetes. Type 1 diabetes (juvenile-onset) occurs when the beta cells of the pancreas become unable to produce insulin. Type 1 diabetes is thought to have an autoimmune component to it, as the body can produce antibodies against the pancreatic beta cells resulting in an inability to produce insulin. Type 1 diabetics need to be treated with insulin in order to control their blood sugar.

Type 2 diabetes is often referred to as adult-onset diabetes. Type 2 diabetes is responsible for 90-95% of all the diagnoses of diabetes. In Type 2 diabetes, the beta cells of the pancreas are usually producing adequate or even large amounts of insulin. However, the insulin is not able to properly control the blood sugar because the insulin receptors are not able to respond appropriately to insulin. When the insulin receptors become resistant to insulin, it is referred to as insulin resistance. The end result is an elevated blood sugar. Type 2 diabetes is associated with obesity, older age, family history of diabetes, as well as physical inactivity. Certain ethnic groups are at an increased risk for type 2 diabetes including African Americans, Hispanic Americans, Asian Americans, and American Indians. The remainder of this chapter will focus on type 2 diabetes. For the remainder of the chapter, when I use the term 'diabetes', I will be referring to type 2 diabetes.

WHAT CAUSES DIABETES?

Does elevated blood sugar cause diabetes? The answer is no. Elevated blood sugar is the marker needed to confirm the diagnosis of diabetes, but it does not cause it. Although the exact cause of type 2 diabetes is not known, there are many underlying factors that are directly related to causing diabetes, as shown in Table 1.

TABLE 1: UNDERLYING FACTORS CAUSING DIABETES

- Eating a diet high in refined sugars
- Genetic predisposition
- Insulin resistance
- Obesity
- Old age

That is not to say that everyone who eats a diet high in refined sugars or who is obese will develop diabetes. Clearly, there are genetic as well as other factors predisposing some to developing diabetes. But, there is no doubt that we have an epidemic of diabetes being caused, in large part, by the above items.

Most of the factors listed above can be influenced by lifestyle changes (except older age and genetic predisposition). My clinical experience has clearly shown that changing the lifestyle factors predisposing one to becoming diabetic is the most important therapy anyone can do to not only prevent, but treat diabetes. This idea will be discussed further at the end of the chapter.

INSULIN RESISTANCE

As previously mentioned, insulin resistance occurs when the body's insulin receptors lose their sensitivity to insulin. This is the most common problem with diabetics and is thought to be the underlying cause of diabetes for the vast majority suffering from it. The end result of insulin resistance is elevated blood sugar, as the cells cannot respond appropriately to insulin.

The human body has been designed with many checks and balances in order to maintain a steady state, or homeostasis. In the case of blood sugar, we function optimally when our blood sugar is less than 100mg/dl. If the body senses blood sugar rising, the beta cells of the pancreas will be signaled, resulting in increased insulin production. This is the normal response of the body to maintaining homeostasis with blood sugar (i.e., keeping blood sugar less than 100mg/dl).

Type 2 diabetics typically suffer from insulin resistance. In the early stages of the illness, they are producing adequate or excess amounts of insulin in order to try and keep blood sugar below 100mg/dl. However, in this case, the usual insulin amounts are unsuccessful at maintaining blood sugar at less than 100mg/dl. The end result is a gradually rising blood sugar and more insulin being released from the beta cells of the pancreas.

As the situation worsens, more and more insulin is produced from the pancreas. Over time, the beta cells of the pancreas will fatigue until the pancreas is unable to produce any more insulin. In the latter stages of diabetes, insulin production will decline and blood sugar will rise. The time to treat type 2 diabetes is before the pancreas becomes fatigued. Once the pancreas stops its production of insulin, the appropriate life-saving treatment will be administering exogenous insulin via shots. Generally, insulin shots will have to be maintained for life.

What causes insulin resistance? There are many causes including: inflammation, obesity (especially abdominal obesity), eating a diet consisting of too many refined foods and sugars (the standard American diet), increased fructose (as well as high fructose corn syrup), high insulin levels, nutrient depletion including vitamin D deficiency, physical inactivity, some medications (e.g., Provera and high steroid doses), poor genetics, and stress.

The good news about insulin resistance is that, in the mid to early stages, it is amenable to treatment. In fact, with a few lifestyle changes, it is easily treated.

CONVENTIONAL MEDICINE'S TREATMENT OF DIABETES: INEFFECTIVE DRUGS

So, how does conventional medicine approach the treatment of diabetes? As previously mentioned, those with type 1 diabetes must be treated with insulin to properly control their blood sugar. Insulin is the proper treatment for type 1 diabetics. The remainder of this discussion pertains to type 2 diabetes only. Any further mention of diabetes will refer to type 2 diabetes unless stated otherwise.

Diabetics are usually treated with oral diabetic medications. These medications have various modes of action, but they generally work by increasing insulin secretion or improving the response of the insulin receptors. This chapter will discuss these various medications and their effects in the body. However, please keep in mind that for the majority of those with type 2 diabetes, they can be effectively treated with lifestyle changes including eating a healthy diet, correcting nutrient deficiencies, exercising, and detoxifying. These items will be discussed near the end of the chapter.

When I lecture to physicians about a particular drug therapy, I make a point of discussing the mode of action of the drug. A drug therapy should treat the underlying cause of the illness for which the drug is being prescribed. Unfortunately, the conventional approach to type 2 diabetes does not treat the underlying cause of the illness. In fact, many of these therapies can actually worsen the illness over time.

Once a diagnosis of type 2 diabetes is made, a conventional physician will probably tell the patient to eat a "diabetic diet" as prescribed by the American Diabetic Association (ADA). Although there is some good information in the ADA's diet plan, it contains so much misinformation that it is best avoided. Diet recommendations for avoiding and treating diabetes will be available at the end of the chapter. Besides the dietary recommendations, a conventional physician will, no doubt, recommend using an oral diabetic medication.

There are different classes of these medications and I will discuss them below. Each class of medication has been shown to lower blood glucose levels in type 2 diabetics. However, each class of medication has been shown to have severe adverse effects and none of the medications effectively addresses the underlying cause of type 2 diabetes. In fact, I will show you that the mode of action of many of these medications actually worsens the illness. Furthermore, every one of the medications is associated with severe adverse reactions. If the medications don't address the underlying cause of the illness, then why should they be the primary therapy prescribed for diabetes?

ORAL ANTIDIABETIC DRUGS

Oral anti-diabetic drugs have been used for over 40 years. Presently, there are many different classes of medications to treat diabetes. I will discuss the most commonly prescribed medications.

All of the oral medications to treat diabetes work to lower blood sugar. However, each class of drugs works by a different mechanism in order to accomplish this. However, I will show you their mechanism of action does not treat the underlying cause of diabetes. If these drugs (or any other drugs for that matter) do not treat the underlying cause of the illness, then I feel they should not be used as a primary treatment modality. At the end of this chapter, I will show you safe and simple ways to make lifestyle changes which do treat the underlying causes of diabetes.

What are the problems with type 2 diabetic drugs? Over 40 years of their use has produced numerous studies on these medications. These studies report consistent findings; an increased heart attack rate and an increased rate of death in those taking type 2 diabetes medications. These increases have been found to occur in every class of type 2 diabetic medication used. Unfortunately, each drug is associated with severe adverse effects which may actually worsen the prognosis of the illness.

FIRST TRIAL OF ORAL DIABETIC AGENTS: INCREASED MORTALITY FROM CARDIOVASCULAR DISEASE

In 1969, the first large trial of oral diabetic agents was undertaken-- the University Group Diabetes Program.   It was a multicenter study designed to evaluate the effects of various diabetic medications on vascular compilations in patients with asymptomatic diabetes. The two drugs studied were Phenformin and Orinase.   Phenformin is part of the class of diabetic medications known as biguanides.   Orinase is a sulfonlylurea drug.

I know my description of these mechanisms of action may make you cross your eyes and become drowsy, but just stay with me and it will all make sense.

These drugs work by completely different mechanisms. Biguanides (Metformin is the present-day biguanide) works by decreasing liver glucose production, increasing insulin sensitivity, and increasing fatty acid oxidation. Sulfonylureas (e.g., Glipizide, and Glyburide are present-day medications) work by binding to specific receptors in the cell membrane of the pancreas (ATP-dependant K^+ channel) which results in increased secretion of insulin from the pancreas.

Keep in mind the two drugs studied had totally different mechanisms of action. The first major study of an oral type 2 diabetic medication was reported in 1971. This study had to be halted two years early due to adverse effects of the oral medications. One arm of the study found that, compared to placebo, Phenformin was found to be responsible for a 400% increase (absolute risk 9.6%) in cardiovascular death rate and a 38% increase in death from any cause.[6] For every 10 people treated with this drug, there was approximately one death (cardiovascular death). A few years later, phenformin was removed from the market after it was established to cause lactic acidosis in diabetic patients with renal failure.

Another arm of the study found that, compared to placebo, Orinase was responsible for a 260% increase (absolute risk 7.8%) in cardiovascular death rate and a 44% increase in death from any cause.[7] For every 13 people treated with Orinase, there was one death (cardiovascular death). Orinase is still available as generic tolbutamide.

WHAT ABOUT THE NEWER DRUGS?

In 1971, Orinase was a first-generation sulfonylurea medication. Presently there are second-generation sulfonylurea medications for use in type 2 diabetes: Glyburide (Diabeta, Glucovance, Glynase, and Micronase) and Glipizide (Glipizide ER, Glipizide, Glucotrol, Glucotrol XL, and Metaglip). These are two widely prescribed categories of second generation sulfonylureas. These drugs cost anywhere from $10 to $100 per month depending on brand name versus generic equivalents. These drugs cost consumers billions of dollars per year.

What are the side effects of these drugs? If you look at the Physician's Desk Reference (PDR), the reported side effects of each of these drugs includes increased risk of cardiovascular mortality. Diabetic patients die from cardiovascular mortality at much higher rates than any other cause of death. Perhaps it would be wise to reconsider using a class of drugs (e.g.., sulfonylureas) that is associated with a higher rate of cardiovascular mortality.

HOW ABOUT METFORMIN?

Metformin (ActoPlus, Actoplus, Avandamet, Glucophage, Glucovance, Prandimet and Riomet) is the most widely prescribed drug for diabetes in the U.S. In 2006, there were over 35 million prescriptions written for it.[8] What are the reported side effects from Metformin? Adverse effects include lactic acidosis (rare), increased risk of renal dysfunction with increasing age, diabetes, congestive heart failure, and other conditions with risk of hypoperfusion. Furthermore, Metformin has been shown to decrease vitamin B12 levels. There are other warnings about Metformin listed in the PDR as well.

WHAT ABOUT THE LATEST DRUGS?

Avandia is part of the thiazolidinediones class of diabetic medications. Actos and Rezulin are also part of this class of diabetic drugs. Avandia's sales peaked at $2.5 billion in 2006. It works by binding to certain cellular receptors (peroxisome-activated receptors) and is thought to decrease insulin resistance.

Avandia, like all of the diabetic drugs, does lower blood sugar. But, similar to the other diabetic medications, a meta-analysis of 42 studies found that there was a 43% increased risk of heart attack and a 64% increased risk of death from cardiovascular causes in subjects treated with Avandia as compared to those treated with a placebo.[9]

This class of medications (e.g., Avandia, Actos, and Rezulin) has also been found to be associated with a 260% increased risk of diabetic macular edema, a condition that can result in blindness.[10] [11]

THE STRAW THAT SHOULD BREAK THE CAMEL'S BACK

Remember, the first study showing increases in heart attacks and deaths with the use of type 2 diabetic medications was reported nearly 40 years ago. The ACCORD study was reported in 2008 and continued to show increased mortality in those that used the newer type 2 diabetic medications.[12]

The ACCORD study looked at 10,251 patients in order to determine whether intensive therapy to tightly control blood sugar would reduce cardiovascular deaths in patients with type 2 diabetes. Intensive therapy patients were prescribed significantly more type 2 diabetic medications as compared to those given standard therapy (less stringent blood sugar control). The results of the study found that those given more drugs achieved lower blood sugar readings. However, the authors also found that the intensive therapy patients (those treated with more diabetic drugs) had a 22% increase in death rate. Furthermore, the intensive therapy group had more episodes of hypoglycemia, fluid retention, and weight gain. Perhaps other means should be employed to treat type 2 diabetes.

WHY DO THE TYPE 2 DIABETIC MEDICATIONS CAUSE SO MANY PROBLEMS?

The reason that these medications cause so many problems is that the mechanism of action of these drugs does not address the underlying cause of type 2 diabetes. Furthermore, these drugs disrupt the normal biochemical pathways in the body by poisoning enzymes. I have been lecturing to doctors and laypeople alike preaching the importance of treating the underlying cause of an illness.

The mechanism of action of the most popular diabetes medications primarily treats the symptoms of the illness (high blood sugar) and not the causes (obesity, inactivity, poor diet, etc.). Only treating the symptoms of the illness is bound to allow the progression of the illness to proceed. Furthermore, disrupting normal physiology with foreign substances (e.g., pharmacologic agents) is a recipe for poor long-term outcomes, as shown with many of these diabetes studies.

TYPE 2 DIABETIC MEDICATIONS: BEST AVOIDED

By now, hopefully you are asking yourself, "Why should anyone take these medications?" The answer is that these medications should only be used as a last resort, if used at all. Over 40 years of research has shown these drugs to be a failure in reversing diabetes and the cause of too many adverse effects. Nearly every one of these drugs significantly increases the risk of cardiovascular disease—the same problem that occurs with diabetes itself. "Primum non nocere" (First, not to harm) should be remembered.

HOW SHOULD TYPE 2 DIABETES BE TREATED? LIFESTYLE CHANGES

So, if type 2 diabetic medications are not the best choice for treating diabetes, how should it be treated?

To formulate an effective treatment plan, you have to research the underlying cause of an illness and develop that treatment plan which addresses the cause.

There is no question in my mind that the major focus in treating and avoiding type 2 diabetes has to be lifestyle changes. Researchers have stated, "Although it is widely believed that type 2 diabetes mellitus is the result of a complex interplay between genetic and environmental factors, compelling evidence from epidemiologic studies indicates that the current worldwide diabetes epidemic is largely due to changes in diet and lifestyle. Prospective cohort studies and randomized clinical trials have demonstrated that type 2 diabetes can be prevented largely through moderate diet and lifestyle modifications."[13]

Losing weight is number one on the list. Americans are the heaviest people on the planet. An estimated 66% of adults in the United States are overweight or obese. [14] Over one-third of adult Americans are obese (35.6% in 2006). Obesity is also affecting children and adolescents—16.3% of those aged 2-19 are considered obese.[15]

There is no doubt that being overweight or obese is the main underlying risk factor for developing type 2 diabetes. Excess fat can result in insulin receptors developing an inability to properly respond to glucose and can lead to insulin resistance.

HOW DO YOU MAKE INSULIN RECEPTORS WORK BETTER?

The answer to the above question is simple; lose weight and exercise. The connection between obesity and the development of type 2 diabetes is very strong and weight loss has been shown to improve all diabetic parameters.

Researchers reported that for overweight individuals, every kg (2.2 pounds) of weight loss over 10 years was associated with a 33% lower risk of diabetes in the subsequent 10 years. These same researchers concluded that, "Weight gain was associated with substantially increased risk of diabetes among overweight adults, and even modest weight loss was associated with significantly reduced diabetes risk. Minor weight reductions may have major beneficial effects on subsequent diabetes risk in overweight adults at high risk of developing diabetes." [16]

Furthermore, research has clearly shown the benefit of exercise in helping insulin receptors improve their function. Exercise is a must for those with diabetes or prediabetes. More about exercise can be found later in this chapter.

OBESITY=INSULIN RESISTANCE

How does obesity relate to the development of diabetes? Insulin resistance is much more common in obesity due to the adipose (fat) tissue's ability to produce inflammation. Researchers hypothesize that it is the inflammation from the fat tissue that is the underlying factor responsible for insulin resistance. [17] [18] Specifically, in obesity, the white adipose tissue is infiltrated by macrophages (white blood cells) which activate locally produced inflammatory cells.

How can you modify this inflammation? Eating foods that promote inflammation will worsen the condition and conversely, eating healthy foods that have anti-inflammatory properties will help this condition.

FOOD: INFLAMMATORY VERSUS ANTI-INFLAMMATORY

Food that promotes inflammation includes food made from refined products such as refined sugar, flour, and salt. Refined food products generally are lacking in vital nutrients such as vitamins, minerals, and enzymes. Examples of refined foods include white bread, chips, pretzels, candy, pasta, and boxed cold cereal. Furthermore, most refined food products contain high fructose corn syrup (refined sugar). During digestion, these refined items, lacking vital nutrients, result in wide blood sugar swings. In a large number of people, the continual ingestion of these items results in a depleted body, blood sugar dysregulation, and diabetes. I have no doubt that the diabetes epidemic we are currently seeing is due, in large part, to the ingestion of too many refined food products.

The glycemic index is a classification of carbohydrates based on how quickly the food is metabolized into glucose. Eating foods with a low glycemic index is beneficial for everyone and helps to prevent diabetes. Examples of low glycemic foods include apples, grapefruit, and green vegetables. The glycemic index can be a good guide to use to help you decide if it is wise to eat a particular food. The glycemic index and other healthy food recommendations can be found in my book, **_The Guide to Healthy Eating._**

Eating unrefined, healthy food products can have an anti-inflammatory effect in the body. Unrefined, healthy food products, such as fruits, vegetables, nuts, beans, seeds, fish (wild), and eggs (from organic sources) can have anti-inflammatory effects in the body. These healthy foods contain naturally occurring vitamins, minerals, protein, fat, and enzymes which provide the body with the basic raw materials it needs to promote health.

EXERCISE AND DIABETES

There is no question that regular exercise can benefit every one of us. There is an overwhelmingly large amount of evidence that individuals who maintain a more physically active lifestyle are much less likely to develop diabetes.

Research has shown that as little as 30 minutes of exercise per day can dramatically increase blood sugar control. Researchers have reported that, "...epidemiological studies indicate that individuals who maintain a physically active lifestyle are much less likely to develop impaired glucose tolerance and non-insulin-dependent diabetes mellitus (NIDDM). Moreover, it was found that the protective effect of physical activity was strongest for individuals at highest risk of developing diabetes."[19]

Regular exercise has been shown to result in a loss of fat from the central regions of the body. [20] As previously explained, the reduction of abdominal fat will help reduce the inflammatory cells responsible for causing insulin resistance and diabetes.

Exercise does not have to be painful. If you are not used to exercise, I suggest starting slow—walking for example. If you cannot do 30 minutes of exercise, begin with five minutes and gradually build yourself up. It may take some time, but the effort is worth it.

HORMONES AND DIABETES

My clinical experience has shown a direct correlation between hormone dysregulation and diabetes. In nearly all diabetics, I have found that adrenal and thyroid hormones are imbalanced. I have treated many diabetic patients with bioidentical, natural hormones and have seen positive benefits on their ability to lose weight and optimize blood sugar when the hormonal system is properly balanced.

The thyroid gland is the main endocrine gland that is responsible for regulating the metabolism of the body. Hypothyroidism, or an underactive thyroid gland, is responsible for a sluggish metabolism which can promote weight gain and diabetes. Approximately 40% of the population may have an undiagnosed, abnormal thyroid problem. Correcting a thyroid problem with the use of a holistic approach has proven to be successful at helping diabetic patients overcome their illness. More information about the thyroid gland can be found in my book, ***Overcoming Thyroid Disorders, 2nd Edition.***

The adrenal glands are responsible for producing hormones which help regulate blood sugar. DHEA is an adrenal hormone that has been shown to be an effective weight management tool by increasing the oxidation of fatty acids. Furthermore researchers found that, compared to a placebo, women experienced a 10% decline in overall abdominal fat with the use of DHEA. Men experienced a 7.4% decline in abdominal fat.[21]

Other hormones that help improve blood sugar regulation include natural testosterone, pregnenolone, natural progesterone, human growth hormone, and natural hydrocortisone. More information on natural, bioidentical hormones can be found in my book, ***The Miracle of Natural Hormones, 3rd Edition.***

I have found it nearly impossible to help a diabetic patient come off medication if the hormonal system is in disarray. Every diabetic patient needs a full hormonal evaluation by a doctor skilled in the use of natural, bioidentical hormones.

SUPPLEMENTS AND DIABETES

Over 17 years of diagnosing and treating diabetics has convinced me of the importance of properly balancing supplements in a diabetic patient. Diabetic patients are notoriously deficient in many important nutrients which provide the body with the raw materials necessary for optimizing blood sugar. In fact, I have yet to see a new diabetic patient not have multiple nutrient deficiencies.

Two of the most common nutrients deficient in diabetic patients are magnesium and iodine. Magnesium is a mineral that is responsible for catalyzing hundreds of reactions in the body. Researchers have identified a link with magnesium deficiency and diabetes as well as insulin resistance. Low magnesium levels have been reported in diabetic patients.[22] A study of over 120,000 subjects found a significant risk of diabetes in subjects with the lowest magnesium levels.[23] Nearly every diabetic patient I have tested over the last 17 years has had a significantly low magnesium level. Magnesium is found in nuts, cocoa, tea, and green, leafy vegetables. Magnesium supplements are widely available. I suggest getting your red blood cell magnesium levels checked before beginning supplementation. Usual doses of magnesium range from 100-400mg/day.

Iodine deficiency is occurring at epidemic rates. My experience has shown that over 95% of 4,000 patients have tested significantly low in iodine. Iodine helps regulate the thyroid gland. It is impossible to have optimal thyroid function when iodine deficiency is present. Iodine (and thyroid hormone) in rats was shown to decrease the incidence of diabetes.[24]

I have found that type 2 diabetic patients can often stop their oral medications after iodine supplementation, as their blood sugar dramatically improves. For those patients treated with insulin, I have been able to lower insulin dosages in nearly every patient treated with iodine. My colleague, Dr. Jorge Flechas has reported similar findings with iodine supplementation in diabetics.

OTHER NUTRIENTS IN DIABETES

There are many other nutrients important for supplying diabetic patients with the necessary raw materials to help them overcome their illness. These nutrients include: chromium, zinc, lipoic acid, vanadium, Vitamins B1, B2, B3, B5, and B6, as well as folic acid, and cinnamon bark. I helped formulate two supplements, Glucontrol and ZensusLean, which I have found very effective for diabetic patients. These products can be found at www.purezenhealth.com or by calling 1-877-898-7873 (For disclosure purposes, I am an owner of PureZenhealth.com).

FINAL THOUGHTS

Unfortunately, diabetes is a common illness in the United States. Conventional medicine's reliance on using oral medications to treat type 2 diabetes has been a disaster. Type 2 diabetes is not occurring at epidemic rates because we have a deficiency of oral medications to treat it. It is occurring because of poor lifestyle choices—unhealthy diets, nutrient depletion and hormonal dysregulation. My experience has been clear; correcting these underlying problems has proven successful at treating type 2 diabetes.

If you are on a type 2 diabetic medication, I do not suggest you stop taking your medication. The best results are achieved by working with a health care provider knowledgeable about how to use natural therapies to treat diabetes. If you are newly diagnosed with type 2 diabetes, look at your lifestyle choices and see if they can be modified to provide you with the best chance to overcome this serious illness.

Diabetes does not have to be a terrible, downward-spiraling illness. It can be properly managed and controlled by following the steps outlined in this chapter.

[1] American Diabetes Assoc. Accessed at www.diabetes.org/about-diabetes.jsp. 4.11.09

[2] FP News. 3.1.09. p. 10

[3] Diabetes Care. 2009;32:287

[4] Diabetes Care. Vol. 31, N. 3. March, 2008. 596

[5] American Diabetes Assoc. IBID. 4.11.09

[6] JAMA. 8.9.71. Vol 217. No. 6 p. 777-84

[7] Diabetes. 19(suppl 2): 789-830. 1970

[8] *Drug Topics* (March 5, 2007

[9] N.Eng. J. of Med. Vol 356:N. 24; June, 2007. 2457-2471.

[10] FP News. 3.1.09

[11] Am.J. Opth. 2009 (doi:10.1016/j.ajo.2008.10.016)

[12] NEJM. Vol. 358; n. 24. June 12, 2008. 2545-2559

[13] An. Rev. of Pub. Health. VOl. 26:445-467. 2005

[14] From: cdc.gov. http://www.cdc.gov/nchs/data/hus/hus08.pdf#075. Accessed 4.18.09

[15] CDC.gov. http://www.cdc.gov/nccdphp/dnpa/obesity/. Accessed 4.18.09

[16] Journal of Epidemiology and Community Health 2000;**54**:596-602

[17] Gerontology. 2009 Apr 8. [Epub ahead of print]

[18] Eur Cytokine Netw. 2006 Mar;17(1):4-12

[19] Sports Med. 1997. Nov;24(5):321-36

[20] Sports Med. 1997. IBID.

[21] JAMA. Nov. 10, 2004;292:2243-2248

[22] Diabetologia. 1993. 36:767

[23] Diabetes Care. 27:134-40, 2004

[24] Autoimmunity. 2009. Feb;42(2):131-8

Chapter 5

Osteoporosis Drugs

INTRODUCTION

According to the National Institutes of Health (NIH), osteoporosis is defined as a skeletal disorder characterized by compromised bone strength predisposing one to an increased risk of fracture.[1] If you listen to the media, mainstream medical organizations, and Big Pharma you would assume that <u>all</u> post-menopausal women as well as many younger women and older men are at a significant risk for osteoporosis.

The NIH states that osteoporosis is a "major threat to Americans". The NIH estimates that 44 million Americans, or 55% of those older than 55 years of age, are at a significantly increased risk of osteoporosis. Furthermore, 10 million Americans are estimated to have osteoporosis and approximately 34 million more have low bone mass which indicates a risk for osteoporosis. Of those with osteoporosis, 80% are women and 20% are men. Four out of ten white women age 50 and older will experience a fracture in their lifetime.[2] The surgeon general of the U.S. claims that osteoporosis is responsible for more than 1.5 million fractures annually in the U.S. including:[3]

- 300,000 hip fractures

- 700,000 vertebral fractures

- 250,000 wrist fractures

- 300,000 fractures at other sites

Osteoporotic fracture-associated costs are expected to rise by 49% over the next 20 years to 25.3 billion dollars.[4]

There is no question that osteoporosis is a serious illness. For someone who has suffered numerous fractures and has a hunched-over posture (dowager's hump), osteoporosis can be devastating. The risk of mortality is 2.8-4 times greater among hip fracture patients as compared to similar aged individuals without a hip fracture.[5]

WHAT IS OSTEOPOROSIS?

Osteoporosis is presently defined as a disease characterized by low bone mass and structural deterioration of bone tissue. This leads to bone fragility and an increased susceptibility to fractures, especially of the hip, spine, and wrist.[6] In other words, bones have become thin, weak, and brittle and are more likely to fracture.

A close reading of the above-mentioned definition for osteoporosis shows that osteoporosis is much more than just decreased bone density. Most doctors, lay-people, and the media are under the mistaken assumption that osteoporosis is solely due to decreased bone mineral density. It is a mistake to assume that osteoporosis=decreased bone density.

The structural deterioration of the bone is a complex subject that relates to the architecture of the bone. Bone is made up of minerals, collagen, and protein. Deficiencies of any of these building blocks will lead to weakened bones and an increased risk of fracture.

Bone density declines naturally in everybody as they age. If you want to maximize the number of people diagnosed with osteoporosis, defining the illness solely in terms of bone density makes sense. However, this narrow definition gives little information on the most important question: who will suffer fractures of the bones in the future? I will show you in this chapter, that the great majority of individuals will never fracture a bone as a result of the natural age-related decline in bone mineral density. Furthermore, sustaining a fracture does not necessarily mean that there is osteoporosis present. A bone will fracture, even in a young, healthy person if there is enough force applied to that bone.

This chapter will show you that lowered bone density is only one of many factors that make up osteoporosis. An inadequate diet, which results in vitamin and mineral deficiencies, can also lead to osteoporosis. In addition, inactivity can contribute to weakened, osteoporotic bones. There are multiple factors that can lead to osteoporosis.

WHAT ARE BONES MADE OF?

The bones provide the structural function for the body. They allow us to stand up against gravity. Bone strength is, in part, genetically determined as well as environmentally determined. Some people are born with errors in their genes that result in the formation of weak bones. Osteogenesis imperfecta is a genetic disorder characterized by bones that break easily, often from little or no apparent cause. Osteogenesis imperfecta can result in a person having just a few or as many as several hundred fractures in a lifetime. Approximately 20-50,000 people are affected with osteogenesis imperfecta in the United States.

In terms of the environment, stronger bones will be present if the bones are used. Weight bearing and exercise are two ways to ensure strong bones. On the other hand, inactivity can result in weaker bones. Furthermore, ensuring a good diet which provides all the nutrients necessary for forming and maintaining strong bones is essential. Eating poor-quality food lacking basic vitamins and minerals is more likely to lead to the formation of weak bones and accelerate bone loss.

The bones are the main storage sites of many (if not most) of the essential minerals for the body. Bones contain the largest amounts of calcium and phosphorus found in the body.

Adequate amounts of calcium and phosphorus are necessary for a wide range of functions in the body including maintaining the optimal functioning of the organs as well as the nervous system. Examples of other minerals found in high amounts in bones are listed in Table 1 below.

TABLE 1: EXAMPLES OF MINERALS FOUND IN HIGH CONCENTRATION IN BONES
Boron
Calcium
Chromium
Copper
Iron
Magnesium
Manganese
Phosphorus
Silica
Strontium
Sulfur
Zinc

As previously mentioned, bones are made up of many different substances including minerals, protein, and collagen. Adequate amounts of these substances are necessary for proper bone formation. As would be expected, the consequence of an inadequate diet resulting in nutritional deficiencies will be suboptimal bone formation and weak, fragile bones.

Many different counter-regulatory mechanisms are present in the body to ensure that calcium and phosphorus are absorbed and adequate amounts are transported to the bones for storage. Vitamin D is one example. Adequate Vitamin D levels help the body absorb calcium from the diet and transport it to the bones for storage. Parathyroid hormone also helps regulate this process. More about these and other regulatory mechanisms will be discussed later in this chapter.

From the beginning of life until the end, the bones are constantly being modified. Healthy bones undergo a process called remodeling whereby old or damaged bone is removed and new bone is produced to take its place. Remodeling of bone occurs throughout life. In fact, in a healthy situation, most of the adult bone is completely replaced every ten years.

The remodeling process is governed by specialized cells in the bones known as osteoclasts and osteoblasts. It is the crucial interaction between these two bone cells that determines whether we will have healthy or diseased bones.

Major Bone Cells Responsible for Bone Health

Osteoclasts: Remove bone   Bone Resorption
Osteoblasts: Lay down new bone   Remodeling Bone

Osteoclasts remove bone by dissolving the mineral matrix that makes up bone. They are derived from the same cells in our bone marrow that produce white blood cells. After the poor quality bone is removed by the osteoclasts, the osteoclasts die and lay down a protein mix that helps to stimulate the osteoblasts to help make new bone and finish the job.

Osteoblasts are often found in the bone cells that are unearthed by the osteoclasts. These cells are responsible for laying down new bone. As the osteoblasts lay down new bone, the healing process of the injured bone is completed.

THE RELATIONSHIP BETWEEN OSTEOCLASTS AND OSTEOBLASTS

In order to have the healthiest, strongest bone possible, it is important to ensure that both of the bone cells—osteoclasts and osteoblasts—are doing their respective jobs. If the osteoclasts are overactive, too much bone may be broken down. Paget's disease and hyperparathyroidism are examples of illnesses that are caused by excessive bone breakdown by osteoclasts.

If the osteoblasts are not laying down enough good quality bone, bone disease and bone problems will develop. Osteogenesis imperfecta is an example of an osteoporotic condition whereby osteoblasts will not function optimally and will not lay down the right matrix to form healthy strong bones.

Osteoblastic function is also impaired with excess steroid use or excess production of hydrocortisone by the adrenal glands.

In order to make strong bone, we need both osteoblasts and osteoclasts to be optimally functioning. Let's take a closer look at the osteoblasts and osteoclasts.

OSTEOBLASTS

Osteoblasts are found throughout the bones, but predominately on the surface of the bones. The osteoblasts lay down a matrix that includes calcium and phosphorus. Furthermore, collagen is produced by these cells which gives bone the strength it needs. When there are mechanical stresses to the bone as in an injury or normal wear-and-tear, the osteoblasts are stimulated to begin their remodeling process. As previously stated, abnormalities with osteoblasts will lead to weak, brittle, osteoporotic bone.

OSTEOCLASTS

Osteoclasts are responsible for removing bone. This process is known as bone resorption. Osteoclasts are derived from the same precursor cells in the bone marrow that produce white blood cells.[7] Consequently, drugs or conditions that inhibit white blood cell formation may adversely affect bone resorption.

Osteoclasts remove bone by releasing chemicals that disrupt the collagen matrix and dissolving the minerals which form the bone. This is done with the use of hydrogen ions. In a healthy body, osteoclasts have a programmed cell death that controls their activity. In other words, after their job is done, the osteoclasts die.

If osteoclastic activity is excessive, too much bone may be broken down leading to brittle, weak, osteoporotic bone. As previously mentioned, examples of illnesses that occur with excess osteoclastic activity are Paget's disease and hyperparathyroidism.

PUTTING IT ALL TOGETHER: THE SYMPHONY OF OSTEOBLASTS AND OSTEOCLASTS

What keeps bones healthy? Normal functioning of both osteoblast and osteoclast cells ensures healthy bones. As can be seen from the previous two sections, both osteoblasts and osteoclasts are important cells in the process of maintaining strong, healthy bones. Abnormalities in either cell group can lead to brittle, weak, osteoporotic bones which fracture easily.

Think about our roads. I live in Michigan, where we are exposed to all types of weather extremes—very hot in the summer and excessively cold in the winter. Our roads take the brunt of the weather leaving us Michiganders to navigate all of the potholes. Once in a great while--a very long while--road crews will repair the broken roads. They have two choices:

1.   Spread out a new load of pavement over the existing potholes, or

2.   Break up the pot-holed road down to the base and rebuild it.

It doesn't take rocket science to realize which repair method will last longer and be more successful. Taking away the broken pieces of the road and rebuilding new road will far outlast just paving over what is already broken. When looking at bone remodeling, the same idea applies. It makes more sense to ensure that both osteoblasts and osteoclasts are functioning adequately to not only take away injured, old bone but also to lay down new bone in its place. The road analogy will make more sense when we review how the common osteoporotic drugs such as Fosomax® work.

Just as I wish the Michigan roads were free of potholes, I would like my bones to have the strongest skeleton possible. Optimizing both osteoclast and osteoblast functioning ensures that old, damaged, weak bone will be removed and new, strong bone will be deposited. The optimal functioning of both osteoblasts and osteoclasts ensures that the strongest bones possible are being produced.

WHAT AFFECTS OSTEOCLAST AND OSTEOBLAST FUNCTIONING?

Osteoclasts and osteoblasts are affected both by our genes as well as the environment. Genes control the size and shape of the bones. DNA mutations can result in osteoblasts and/or osteoclasts unable to perform their functions. This leads to weak, brittle, osteoporotic bone. Osteogenesis imperfecta is an example of an illness caused by a genetic defect which leads to extremely weak bones.

Environmental influences can also directly affect bone health or disease. Environmental influences are summarized in Table 2 below.

TABLE 2: ENVIRONMENTAL INFLUENCES ON BONES

Alcohol consumption
Calcium intake
Diet
Lack of exercise
Nutritional status
Phosphorus intake
Smoking
Toxins
Vitamin D status

Exercise has been shown to be a tremendous benefit for the bones. Researchers have shown that exercise has the greatest positive effect on bones during childhood and puberty.

Further research has indicated that young athletes can cut their risk of future fracture by nearly 50% by being active.[8]

Both osteoblasts and osteoclasts respond to many of the environmental influences stated in Table 2. For example, Vitamin D deficiency results in elevated parathyroid hormone levels which can stimulate osteoclastic activity to increase. This will result in bone resorption being increased. Too much bone resorption will result in excess bone breakdown. I see a lot of patients who have a hyperparathyroid condition caused by low Vitamin D levels. Long-term elevated hyperparathyroid levels will lead to weakened bones and an increased risk of fracture. The solution to this problem is easy: supplement with Vitamin D.

Joyce, age 64, was distraught. "I thought I was healthy. I went to my doctor and she ordered a bone mineral density test. When the report came back, she told me I had osteoporosis and that if I didn't do anything about it, I would definitely be at an increased risk of fracturing my bones.   I eat well, exercise, and take my vitamins. I was upset," she said. Joyce was prescribed Fosomax® to treat her osteoporotic condition. When Joyce read the package insert about Fosomax®, she decided not to take it. "There was no way I was going to take that drug. The side effects looked worse than the cure," she said. When I evaluated Joyce, I found that she had a very low Vitamin D level (13 ng/ml) and an elevated parathyroid hormone level (75pg/ml). As previously mentioned, the elevated parathyroid hormone level was due to the low Vitamin D level in her body. Joyce was treated with Vitamin D (5,000Units/day) for three months. At a recheck, her parathyroid level had declined to a normal 30 pg/ml. Joyce was prescribed a holistic treatment program that included correcting vitamin and mineral deficits. A bone mineral density test one year later showed that Joyce's bone mineral density improved by an average of 4%. "I was thrilled. Not only do I feel better, I didn't have to take an expensive drug that has so many side effects," she said.

Joyce's case has been repeated over and over in my practice. Joyce did not have an 'osteoporotic drug deficit'. She had a Vitamin D deficiency that caused an elevated parathyroid hormone level, leading to osteoporosis. When the underlying problem was corrected (Vitamin D deficiency), her bone density test improved.

WHAT ABOUT BONE MINERAL DENSITY TESTING?

As previously mentioned, osteoporosis is presently defined as a disease characterized by low bone mass and structural deterioration of bone tissue, leading to bone fragility and an increased susceptibility to fractures, especially of the hip, spine, and wrist.[9] In other words, bones have become thin, weak, and brittle and are therefore more likely to fracture.

Bone mineral density (BMD) refers to the amount of mineralized tissue in bones in the area scanned. In simpler terms, bone mineral density testing is thought to measure the amount of minerals in the bone.

Dual X-ray Absorptiometry (DXA) testing was developed in the 1980's to quantify bone mineral density. The test was brought to market to help physicians decide which patients may be at an increased risk for osteoporosis. Before BMD testing was available, the diagnosis of osteoporosis was made in people whose bones fractured as a result of minimal impact due to thin, brittle bones.

The normal BMD levels were thought to be the average BMD test of young white women (in their 20's). This is referred to as the 'T-score' on BMD testing.

Osteopenia was defined as a BMD test that is from 1.0-2.5 standard deviations below normal. The lowered BMD test refers to a lowered bone mineral content which is one risk factor for osteoporosis.

The World Health Organization (WHO) released a consensus statement that osteoporosis is defined in the bone mineral density testing as a score that is below 2.5 standard deviations of normal. The WHO warns that for each standard deviation decrease in bone mineral density testing, the future fracture risk doubles.[10]

However, those numbers are misleading. As Gillian Sanson points out in her excellent book, ***The Myth of Osteoporosis,*** "This new {BMD} definition {for diagnosing osteoporosis} meant that millions of women suddenly qualified for diagnosis of a disease for which they had never considered themselves at risk. The 'normal' level is a young person with high bone density. That ensures that a {normal} age-related decrease in bone density is automatically categorized as abnormal."[11]   What the WHO has done is categorize a normal part of aging—bone loss—as a disease requiring the use of an expensive drug.

As Sanson points out, what is less well known about the WHO consensus statement is that the original study that defined osteoporosis as dependant on the BMD test was funded by three major drug companies.[12]   The end-result of this study was that millions of women were now classified as having a disease—osteoporosis—or a pre-disease—osteopenia—that required the long-term use of an expensive prescription medication.   Big Pharma could not have asked for more.

It has become almost gospel that low bone mineral density=osteoporosis. The media, Big Pharma, most mainstream medical groups as well as the WHO, CDC (Center for Disease Control), NIH (National Institutes of Health), and other governmental agencies release report after report touting the efficacy of using BMD tests to diagnose and start treatment for osteopenia/osteoporosis. But is bone mineral testing actually the best test to diagnose osteoporosis?

WHAT DOES BMD TELL US?

That is the million dollar question. A BMD test shows a radiographic view of the density of the bones. It is well known that bones reach their peak mass at young adulthood. As we age, bone density declines like so many other physiologic functions in our bodies. Does the natural, age-related decline of bone mass indicate an illness? Of course not. The bones, like all tissues in our bodies, are not as strong as when we were young. This is a normal part of the aging process.

What is less well publicized is that bone mass varies greatly between ethnic groups, genders, across geographical regions of a country, and even between seasons.[13] Sanson argues that the reference ranges used by BMD testing machines does not take these variations into account.

If BMD declines naturally when we age, is it reasonable to assume that at age 50 your bones should be as dense as they were when you were 25? This is an absurd question. Nothing works as well at age 50 as it did when you were 25. This includes BMD.

Can BMD testing give you an indication of fracture risk? The media, mainstream medical organizations and others would answer with a resounding "YES". However, the research provides a different answer.

DOES BMD TESTING PREDICT FRACTURE RATES?

Preventing fractures is the ultimate goal of any osteoporotic therapy. Can you fracture bones with low BMD? Yes. Can you fracture bones with normal BMD? Of course you can. Does BMD testing predict your future risk for fractures? The surprising answer is no.

Let's look at the National Institute of Health definition of osteoporosis again: Osteoporosis is defined as a skeletal disorder characterized by compromised bone strength predisposing to an increased risk of fracture.[14] This definition states not only compromised bone strength, but an increased risk of fracture. Does BMD testing predict fracture rates? Researchers are divided on how to answer this question.

Many cultures have low BMD but low fracture rates. The Japanese are an example of this. Fracture rates are much lower in Asia, South America and Africa as compared to the United States. In most of these countries, women are not being routinely screened for BMD and treated for low BMD. Remember, you can have thin, strong bones as well as weak, thick bones. BMD testing cannot distinguish between strong and weak bones. Normal age-related bone loss does not increase the risk of fracture.

What is normal age-related bone loss? No one knows the answer to that question. The studies have not been done to determine the definition of normal age-related bone loss. Big Pharma does not want that question answered because it will markedly decrease the number of prescriptions of osteoporosis drugs. At the present time, osteoporotic drugs are recommended for nearly any woman who shows a decline in her BMD testing.

So, does BMD testing predict the risk of fracture? There are arguments for and against BMD being able to predict the risk of fracture. But, there is no consensus. Furthermore, research has not been able to show conclusively that BMD testing can predict the future risk of fracture. Researchers in British Columbia, after a thorough review of the evidence, concluded, "BMD testing is unable to accurately distinguish women at low risk of fracture from those at high risk."[15] Many other researchers have come to a similar conclusion.[16] Bone mineral density testing is one (of many) risk factors for developing osteoporosis. It is in no way the definitive test that determines who will eventually fracture bones. I believe the research has been clear; bone mineral density testing is not accurate enough to predict who will fracture bones in the future.

Many other researchers have come to a similar conclusion. "Bone mineral density testing of healthy women continues to increase, despite widespread discrediting of this test as a valid means to predict fracture risk. BMD testing has grown because it is marketed in ways that draw upon and perpetuate two trends in western popular culture: a) the medical model of the aging female body; and b) the fear of aging with its associated and perpetuated notion that the aging female body is a diseased body."[17]

WHY HAS BMD TEST BEEN SO PROMOTED? CLEVER MARKETING AND MISINFORMATION

So, if BMD testing cannot accurately predict who will fracture, why has the test been so highly promoted? I believe it is due to clever marketing and misinformation. It is similar to the hype that Big Pharma marshaled when it promoted the use of synthetic hormone replacement therapy (HRT) to treat menopausal symptoms, as well as prevent coronary artery disease and osteoporosis. For over 25 years, the media, mainstream medical organizations, and Big Pharma promoted the use of HRT, which became a multi-billion dollar industry. Most physicians bought into the hype and actively promoted HRT to their patients as an effective tool to prevent the ravages of aging. It took 25 years of HRT hype until the accurate information finally came out. HRT did not prevent or treat many of the conditions Big Pharma claimed it treated. In fact, the largest study to look at the effects of HRT therapy, the Women's Health Initiative, found that synthetic HRT therapy resulted in a:[18]

1. 29% increase risk of coronary artery disease.
2. 26% increase in the risk of invasive breast cancer.
3. 41% increase in strokes.
4. 205% increase in Alzheimer's disease.
5. 2,100% increase in blood clots to the lung—pulmonary embolism.

THE LIMITATIONS OF BMD TESTING

BMD testing gives no information about the tensile strength of the bones. It only gives information about the density of bones. As previously stated, you can have strong, thin bones as well as weak, thick bones. If physicians were aware of the limitations of the BMD test, I believe far fewer tests and prescriptions for osteoporotic drugs would be ordered. Physicians need to understand that bone mineral density testing is only one of many risk factors for osteoporosis (see next page). BMD testing has never been shown to predict future fracture risk. Furthermore, if physicians understood the mechanism of how the most prescribed drugs (bisphosphonates) actually work, I believe most physicians would search for other methods to diagnose, prevent, and treat osteoporosis. More information on how osteoporotic drugs work will be found later in this chapter.

TABLE 3: RISK FACTORS FOR OSTEOPOROSIS

Decrease in weight since age 25
Decrease in height since age 25
Greater amount of caffeine intake
Low bone mineral density
Maternal history of hip fracture
Previous hyperthyroidism
Self-rating of health as fair or poor
Spending less than or equal to four hours per day on feet

The incidence of hip fracture was 1.1/1000 women-years among women with not more than two risk factors and normal BMD of the heel for their age.
The incidence of hip fracture was increased to 27/1000 women-years among women with five or more risk factors and lowered BMD of the heel for their age.

WHAT ARE THE RISK FACTORS FOR OSTEOPOROSIS?

There are multiple risk factors for osteoporosis as shown in Table 3. [19] [20] Unfortunately, the media, many physicians and most mainstream medical organizations focus on the BMD test as the sole risk factor for osteoporosis. Increasing BMD has never been conclusively shown to reduce fracture risk. If more attention was paid to identifying and addressing as many of the other risk factors as possible, real progress (with less expense) could be made in treating those with true osteoporosis.

AN IMBALANCED HORMONAL SYSTEM CAN BE A RECIPE FOR OSTEOPOROSIS

One of the most common themes I observe in osteoporotic patients is that their hormonal system is almost always in disarray. Our bones have receptors for hormones throughout their structure. As we age, hormonal levels naturally fall. Although the decline in hormone levels due to aging is not a pathologic process, when this age-related decline is accelerated, the risk for osteoporosis is increased. In other words, maintaining a balanced hormonal system will result in stronger bones.

As I have described in ***The Miracle of Natural Hormones 3rd Edition,*** many hormones have anabolic or tissue rebuilding properties. This tissue-rebuilding effect includes the bones as well as the muscles. Examples of hormones that have anabolic effects are:

1. DHEA
2. Human growth hormone
3. Pregnenolone
4. Testosterone

In the case of either osteopenia or osteoporosis, it is vitally important to ensure a balanced, well-functioning hormonal system. Furthermore, I have found it nearly impossible to reverse osteoporosis without the use of bioidentical, natural hormones.

Other hormones such as bioidentical progesterone and estrogen, are also helpful in preventing and treating osteoporosis.

HORMONAL FACTORS WHICH INCREASE THE RISK FOR OSTEOPOROSIS

Certain hormonal factors can increase the risk for developing osteoporosis. Table 4 below gives the hormonal factors responsible for increasing the risk of developing osteoporosis.

TABLE 4: HORMONAL RISK FACTORS FOR OSTEOPOROSIS
Estrogen deficiency Excess cortisone Hypopituitarism Hyperparathyroidism Medroxyprogesterone acetate (Provera®) Progesterone deficiency Prolactinoma Testosterone deficiency

Provera®, a synthetic progesterone analogue has been shown to cause osteoporosis. In fact, the FDA has issued a 'Black Box' warning on the use of Provera® as its use may actually cause irreversible osteoporosis.[21] As I describe in **_The Miracle of_**

Natural Hormones, 3rd Edition, Provera is a dangerous drug that should not be used for any condition. The FDA should take out of the "Black Box" and remove it from the market. More information about Provera® can be found in Chapter 9.

MEDICATIONS AS A CAUSE OF OSTEOPOROSIS

Through a variety of mechanisms, many medications have been associated with increasing the fracture risk. Some medications cause sedation and can cause balance problems, particularly with the elderly. Antidepressants, sedatives, and sleeping pills fall into this category. Other medications can cause dizziness and unsteadiness. All of these factors can lead to an increased risk of falls and fractures. Table 5 lists some medications associated with an increased risk of bone fractures.

TABLE 5: MEDICATIONS THAT CAN INCREASE THE RISK OF FRACTURES

1. Antacids
2. Anticonvulsant drugs
3. Antidepressants
4. Sedatives (benzodiazepines)
5. Sleeping pills
6. Warfarin (Coumadin®)

Of all the medications listed in Table 5, Coumadin® may be the least known to increase the fracture risk. Coumadin®, used by millions as an anticoagulant, inhibits the synthesis of Vitamin K-dependant clotting factors. In research, Coumadin® has been shown to promote loss, thinning and weakening of bone. Researchers have found that in osteoporotic subjects, Vitamin K levels were found to be 65% lowered as compared to subjects without osteoporosis.[22]

Vitamin K is integral to activating the protein osteocalcin which is essential to calcify and strengthen bones. Inactivated osteocalcin (undercarboxylated osteocalcin) has been associated with high skeletal turnover, low BMD, and increased risk of osteoporotic fracture.[23] Lowered Vitamin K levels have been found in women who have fractured hips as compared to women who did not have hip fractures.[24] Researchers have also reported a 340% increase in vertebral fractures in subjects treated with long-term coumadin.[25]

My colleague, Jonathan Wright, M.D., has "observed decreases in urinary calcium loss (as well as decreases in bone peptide loss) in women after they started taking Vitamin K".[26] I have observed similar results in my patients. I have seen many positive results (via BMD tests, calcium excretion results) when using Vitamin K supplementation.

OTHER RISK FACTORS FOR OSTEOPOROSIS ARE MORE IMPORTANT THAN BMD TESTS

Table 6 lists other miscellaneous risk factors for osteoporosis.[27] Most hip fractures occur after a fall, but most falls (over 99%) do not result in a hip fracture. The NIH has reported that fracture risk is associated with impaired physical functioning such as slow gait speed, impaired cognition, impaired vision, and the presence of environmental hazards such as throw rugs.[28] Many other researchers have concluded that BMD is not the best predictor of hip fractures in the elderly as compared to low body weight, kyphosis, poor circulation in the foot, epilepsy, poor trunk maneuverability, and steroid use. One study concluded that, "A combination of readily obtained risk factors can identify elderly women who will sustain a hip fracture in the next three years more accurately than bone measurements alone in younger women."[29]

Table 6: Miscellaneous Risk Factors for Osteoporosis

1. Being tall at age 25
2. Celiac disease
3. Consumption of dairy products
4. Cystic fibrosis
5. Decreased quadriceps strength (thigh muscles)
6. Excess alcohol use
7. Folic acid deficiency
8. Inflammatory bowel disease
9. Poor nutrition
10. Presence of environmental hazards (tripping)
11. Risk of falls
12. Slow gait speed
13. Vitamin B12 deficiency
14. Vitamin K deficiency

It is clear that the healthier an individual is, the less likely a fracture will occur with a fall. It is important to assess for impaired cognition or vision, environmental hazards, and to make sure good nutrition is followed to help the elderly avoid fractures. A holistic approach accompanying the above mentioned items is more effective to prevent fractures than solely relying on BMD testing. Furthermore, it is a lot less expensive and it makes more sense to assess and intervene with the factors mentioned in Table 6 instead of relying solely on pharmacologic therapy.

CELIAC DISEASE

Celiac disease or sensitivity to the protein gluten, is a major, unrecognized risk factor for osteoporosis. Gluten is the protein found in certain grains such as wheat, rye, and barley. Celiac disease is woefully under diagnosed. It affects nearly one in 133 Americans. Presently 97% of cases of celiac disease go undiagnosed.[30] Every new patient that comes to my office is screened for celiac disease. When celiac disease is diagnosed and treated with a gluten-free diet, bone density almost always improves. Researchers have also documented improved BMD in gluten-sensitive individuals treated with a gluten-free diet.[31]

DOES DAIRY CONSUMPTION PROTECT AGAINST OSTEOPOROSIS?

Special mention must be made of dairy products. Who is not familiar with the commercials of the athletic people with the milk-mustache and the slogan "Got Milk?" The dairy industry would like us to believe that drinking milk gives you strong bones and prevents osteoporosis. However, the research gives a far different picture.

The Harvard Nurses Health Study, which followed more than 75,000 women for 12 years failed to show a protective effect of increased milk consumption on risk of fractures. In addition, this study found that an increased intake of calcium from dairy products was actually associated with a higher fracture risk.[32]

A 10-year study at Penn State found that calcium and dairy intake was not associated with bone gain or bone strength. In this study, only exercise during adolescence was significantly correlated with increased BMD and bone strength.[33]

A review of 58 studies on calcium and dairy consumption concluded that, "Scant evidence supports nutrition guidelines focused specifically on increasing milk or other dairy products for promoting child and adolescent bone mineralization."[34] Another large review (57 studies) found that 71% of the studies showed no benefit from ingesting dairy and 14% of the studies actually showed that diary products weaken bones.[35] Diary products are very allergenic as well. My clinical experience has clearly shown no benefit to bones from those who ingest dairy.

Dairy products preventing osteoporosis is another example of clever marketing and misinformation.

PREVENTING OSTEOPOROSIS: WHO NEEDS TREATMENT?

If you believe Big Pharma, anyone over the age of 50, especially all women, are osteoporotic or osteopenic and in need of expensive drug therapy to prevent them from dying from a fracture. However, it is important to remember: most people will never have an osteoporotic fracture. Furthermore, just because you suffer a fracture does not mean that you have osteoporosis. If the trauma to the bone is of such a strong force, anyone can suffer a fracture. Young people suffer fractures when the force is sufficient to break the bone. Osteoporosis refers to brittle, weakened bones that fracture with minimal impact.

As stated earlier, the current consensus in conventional medicine is to test everyone for their BMD at age 50 and begin drug treatment when the bone density reaches a critical threshold of -2.5 standard deviations as compared to a younger age. Many patients are treated when their bone mineral density test reaches -1.0 standard deviations. Remember, most BMD tests compare your bone age to a young woman in her 20's. Everyone has a lower bone density at age 50 as compared to age 20. Big Pharma would have us all believe that most every woman over 50 years of age should be tested and the majority treated. However, there is little or no scientific data showing this regimen will result in a lowered fracture risk. What this regimen will do is cost a lot of money and give people a lot of adverse side effects.

I feel conventional medicine's approach to diagnosing and treating osteoporosis is much too broad and it does not make sense. Everyone loses bone as they age. If we compared nearly any aging marker, from most hormone levels to skin elasticity, most aging markers decline as we age. This includes bone density.

There is a purpose for BMD testing. It is <u>one of many</u> markers of bone health. Other markers were listed in Table 3 (pg. 123). BMD testing can be used as part of a complete evaluation of a person's health status. This evaluation can include measuring vitamin, mineral, and hormone levels in addition to eliciting a complete dietary history. I do not feel BMD testing should be the sole marker used to determine if one needs to take a life-long expensive medication that is associated with numerous side effects.

It is important for all of us to maintain a healthy lifestyle. A healthy lifestyle, which includes eating nutritious foods, regular exercise, and drinking enough water will help us all achieve our optimum health.

Someone who has suffered numerous fractures due to minimal impact and has other risk factors for osteoporosis will need treatment to help strengthen and repair the bones. What treatments are available? Do these individuals need osteoporotic drugs? Does anyone need osteoporotic drugs?

OSTEOPOROSIS TREATMENT: BISPHOSPHONATES

Who is not aware of the osteoporosis drugs? Television commercials and newspaper ads constantly hammer the message that most post-menopausal women need to be tested for osteoporosis and, if needed, treated with drugs that treat osteoporosis.   Are these drugs truly life-saving?   Are they effective   in   preventing   or   treating   osteoporosis? Bisphosphonates have been used widely for over 12 years. Do these drugs prevent fractures? This section will answer these questions.

The FDA has approved bisphosphonates for treating osteoporosis, osteitis deformans (Paget's disease), bone metastasis, multiple myeloma, and other diseases that have bone fragility as a presenting symptom. Examples of bisphosphonate drugs include Fosomax®, Actonel®, Zometa® and Boniva®.

Bisphosphonates are a class of drugs that inhibit the resorption of bone. Recall from earlier in this chapter, there are two processes to having healthy bones: bone resorption and bone remodeling. Bone resorption is the process whereby old, injured bone is removed and bone remodeling is the process whereby new bone is produced. In more practical terms, old bone is taken away (resorption) and new, strong bone is deposited (remodeling).

Bisphosphonates work by attaching to bone tissue and are absorbed by the osteoclasts. Once absorbed by the osteoclasts, bisphosphonates poison the enzyme farnesyl diphosphate synthase in the HMG-CoA pathway. This results in the death of the osteoclasts.

THE HALF-LIFE OF FOSOMAX: >10 YEARS

The half-life of a drug is the amount of time it takes for 50% of the drug to be eliminated from the body. For comparison, the half-life of estradiol is approximately 1.7 hours.[36] The half-life of progesterone is 5-20 minutes and the half-life of testosterone is 2.1 hours.[37] [38]

Fosomax® was found to have a terminal half-life of greater than 10 years (Greater than 10 years—is it 50 years or 100 years? No one knows.).[39] This means that it takes at least 10 years for one-half of the dose of Fosomax® to break down in the body. This long half-life is unacceptable for any therapy. Once this drug binds to the bone and poisons the osteoclasts, the body has no mechanism to rid itself of the bisphosphonate. This long half-life ensures these drugs will have long-term adverse effects that may not be reversible. Pesticides, heavy metals, and other poisons have a very long half-life in our bodies because we do not have mechanisms to detoxify these items out of our bodies.

Statins (e.g., Lipitor—see Chapter 2) also poison an enzyme in the HMG-CoA pathway, but they do not bind to bone tissue in an appreciable amount. There is some research that claims that statins can increase bone density by poisoning the same enzyme, but this has not been proven.

Poisoning of the osteoclasts disrupts the normal functioning between the osteoblasts and the osteoclasts. The end result with using bisphosphonates is that osteoclastic activity (bone resorption) declines while remodeling (bone deposition) continues. The use of bisphosphonates has been shown to result in an increased bone density. Remember, bone density testing only measures the thickness or density of the bones. An increased bone density does not necessarily mean increased bone strength.

Fosomax® is the most common bisphosphonate used. In 2004, over two million prescriptions for Fosomax® were written which resulted in a revenue of nearly $2,000,000,000.[40] The most common bisphosphonates prescribed today are listed in Table 7 below.

TABLE 7: COMMONLY PRESCRIBED BISPHOSPHONATE DRUGS

Actonel   (Risedronate)
Boniva   (Ibandronate)
Didronel (Etidronate)
Fosomax (Alendronate)
Zometa   (Zoledronate)

DO BISPHOSPHONATES BUILD HEALTHY, STRONG BONES?

Remember, you can't poison a crucial enzyme and expect a good long-term result. Researchers looked at rats that were given Fosomax® after a spinal fusion and bone graft was performed. There was a control group given no therapy, and two treatment groups. One treatment group was given the standard dose of Fosomax® and a second treatment group was treated with a high dose of Fosomax®. X-ray appearance showed improved bone density in both treatment groups. However, at autopsy, both treatment groups were found to have poor quality bone remodeling as well as poor osteoclastic and osteoblastic function.[41]

Another study of rats given bone grafts found that Fosomax® actually inhibited bone graft resorption and incorporation.[42] A similar study in rabbits found that Fosomax inhibits bone fusion.[43] Fosomax®, by poisoning a crucial enzyme in bone metabolism, is bound to inhibit bone healing and normal bone function.

DO BISPHOSPHONATES LOWER FRACTURE RISK?

That is the million dollar question that is yet to be answered. The true question that we should be looking at is: Do the bisphosphonates result in fewer fractures? The research is far from clear on this question.

Unfortunately, we do not have a single test to measure bone strength. As I have stated throughout this book, **you can't poison a crucial enzyme or block an important receptor and expect a good long-term outcome.** Good bone strength is determined by the coordinated activity of both osteoclasts and osteoblasts. In other words, our bones need both remodeling and resorption. Our bones were not designed to have one-half of the rebuilding process (i.e., osteoclastic resorption) poisoned and taken out of the picture. You may get thicker bones with the bisphosphonates, but I doubt that you will get stronger bones. In fact, I feel the long-term use of these medications will cause the opposite situation to occur—it will lead to the formation of poor quality bone. What does the research show?

There are experts on both sides--those that claim that bisphosphonates lower fracture risk and those that claim they do not lower fracture risk. If bisphosphonates do lower fracture risk, that lowered risk is very small—at least according to the research. On the Merck website (www.fosomax.com), there is an ad showing a 51% decline in hip fractures with a three year trial (FIT trial) of Fosomax®. Further investigation into the data showed that of the 2,027 studied, after three years there were 22 fractures in the placebo group (2.2%) and 10 in the Fosomax®

group (1.1%).[44] The absolute risk reduction was 1%. The website used the less accurate relative risk reduction to make the claim of a 50% reduction. On the same web page, Merck claims a 44% reduction in vertebral fractures. Again, a closer look at the data shows that out of 4,134 women studied, 2.1% (43 women) had a vertebral fracture taking Fosomax® as compared to 3.8% (78 women) not taking Fosomax. The most important number to look at is the absolute reduction in vertebral fractures which was 1.7%. I do not feel a 1.7% reduction in fractures is anything to get excited about, especially when the drug is expensive and has multiple adverse effects (see Table 8 pg. 139). I feel there are safer and more effective measures to improve bone strength than taking a drug which poisons a crucial enzyme in the body.

Gillian Sanson states, "If a woman has low bone density (osteopenia), but no previous fractures, her risk for fracture is low."[45] She points out the research that shows a large number of women that need to be treated to prevent one fracture. In the case of osteopenia without a history of fracture, researchers have estimated that 60 women would have to be treated for three years to prevent one vertebral fracture.[46] In women who have osteoporosis with a history of fractures, estimates are that 15 women would need treatment for three years to prevent a single fracture in one of them.[47] Remember, these studies did not look at any other methods of preventing and reversing osteoporosis;

they only focused on drug therapies. I believe there are other options available that make more sense, are significantly less expensive, and have far less adverse side effects as compared to osteoporotic drug therapies. These safer options will be discussed at the end of this chapter.

ADVERSE EFFECTS OF BISPHOSPHONATES

Bisphosphonates have a plethora of adverse effects. In fact, many patients discontinue these drugs because the side effects are so unpleasant. Table 8 provides the most common side effects of the bisphosphonates.

TABLE 8: SIDE EFFECTS OF BISPHOSPHONATES	
Acute-phase reaction	Joint pain
Bone pain	Musculoskeletal pain
Electrolyte disturbance	Nephrotic syndrome
Esophageal erosions	Osteomalacia
Eye inflammation	Osteonecrosis of the jaw
Flu-like symptoms	Seizures
Hyperphosphatemia	Skin rash
Increased PTH	Transient leucopenia
Inflammation	Upset stomach

One of the most common complaints I hear from my patients that take a bisphosphonate drug is burning pain going up the chest. This burning pain is from the direct contact of the drug to the esophagus as well as the drug inducing a generalized inflammatory response in the body (more information on bisphosphonates and inflammation on page 141). One recommendation is to stay upright for one hour after taking the medication. In order to avoid this adverse effect, the best recommendation I can give you is not to take this toxic medication in the first place.

One of the most serious side effects of the bisphosphonates is osteonecrosis of the bone, which I will discuss in the next section. Remember, *you can't poison a crucial enzyme, as bisphosphonates do, and expect a good long-term result.*

BISPHOSPHONATES AND OSTEONECROSIS OF THE JAW

Osteonecrosis of the jaw is sometimes referred to as 'dead jaw'. It refers to a condition in which the bone tissue in the jaw fails to heal after a minor trauma. Reports of osteonecrosis of the jaw have been increasing since the introduction of bisphosphonagte drugs. Symptoms of osteonecrosis include pain, loosening of teeth, and numbness or heaviness of the jaw. There is no known treatment for this condition. Researchers have reported an increased risk of osteonecrosis of the jaw in patients taking bisphosphonate drugs who undergo tooth extractions or dental surgeries.[48] A class–action lawsuit was filed against Merck (Fosomax®) for failing to disclose the side effect of osteonecrosis.

Why would a bisphosphonate drug increase the risk of osteonecrosis? Remember the mechanism of how normal bone function occurs? Osteoclasts are the cells responsible for removing old and injured bone tissue (bone resorption) and osteoblasts are responsible for laying down new bone. If you poison the osteoclasts with a drug such as a bisphosphonate, the healing process will be altered.

Let's take the example of a patient on a bisphosphonate drug that needs a tooth extracted. The extraction process injures the surrounding bone of the jaw. If the healing process has been compromised from the use of a bisphosphonate drug, the body cannot heal the injured bone. The end result may be 'dead jaw' or osteonecrosis. For the patient, it is a devastating outcome, as there is no known cure.

There are many studies which show a correlation between bisphosphonates and osteonecrosis of the jaw.[49] [50] [51] To be fair, there are other studies which do not draw the same conclusion.[52] [53] However, when you use a drug that poisons a crucial enzyme, you will be unable to predict the effects of that drug in the individual.

BISPHOSPHONATES AND INFLAMMATION

Bisphosphonates have been known to activate the inflammatory cascade since 1993.[54] Increased inflammation has been associated with nearly every disease process known. In fact, doctors are routinely checking their patients for inflammation as it has been associated with a markedly increased risk of strokes and heart attacks. Bisphosphonates induce inflammation in the immune system cells—macrophages. In fact, this same inflammatory process has been shown to lead to plaque build-up in the arteries and rupture of arterial plaque which can result in stroke and heart attack.[55]

Other inflammatory problems associated with bisphosphonates include:[56]

1. Acute Polyarthritis[57]
2. Uveitis (eye inflammation)[58]
3. Hepatitis[59]
4. Inflammatory skin reactions[60]
5. Pancreatitis[61]

OTHER MEDICATIONS USED TO TREAT OSTEOPOROSIS

There are other bisphosphonates used to treat osteoporosis such as Actonil®. Since Actonil® has the same mode of action as Fosomax®, it has a similar adverse effect profile. There are also other classes of medications used to treat osteoporosis such as Raloxifene® or Evista®. These drugs are selective estrogen receptor modulators. Both of these medications have serious side effects including increasing the risk of endometrial cancer and blood clots. Forteo® is a synthetic form of parathyroid hormone. Forteo® would make sense in treating osteoporosis if there is a parathyroid hormone deficiency present.

However, there is a black box warning for Forteo® that its use in rats resulted in an elevation of bone cancer--osteosarcoma. When you take into account the side effect profiles of all of these drugs, I believe there are far safer and more effective treatments available (see below).

Although a thorough review of all of the treatments for osteoporosis is beyond this book, it must be kept in mind that osteoporosis is not an illness caused by a drug deficiency. I feel it is a multifactorial problem that can only be thoroughly addressed from a holistic standpoint that takes into account diet and nutrition.

HOW DO YOU PREVENT OSTEOPOROSIS?

The question everyone wants answered is, "How do you prevent osteoporosis?" Osteoporosis can be debilitating when fractures result, especially hip fractures. Hip fractures can be a life-threatening event for an elderly patient. In 2001, hip fractures resulted in 315,000 adult Americans being admitted to hospitals. Over 24% of hip fracture patients over 50-years-old die in the year following their fracture.[62] However, most deaths from hip fractures occur in individuals who also have a major health disorder. Gillian Sanson, author of *The Myth of Osteoporosis* claims, "For those in good health prior to a hip fracture, the injury rarely leads to death."[63]

The best way to prevent osteoporosis is to lead a healthy lifestyle. This healthy lifestyle includes getting regular exercise, eating healthy food, drinking adequate amounts of water, ensuring a balanced hormonal system, and taking appropriate vitamins and minerals that help to make strong bones. The next several sections will give you a healthy road map to maintaining your healthiest bone.

HOW TO MAINTAIN HEALTHY BONES

1. MAINTAIN A NEUTRAL pH

Perhaps the most important single thing you can do to help prevent osteoporosis is to maintain a neutral pH. All functions of our body perform optimally when the pH is around 7.2. The Standard American Diet (SAD), with its over-reliance on refined, devitalized foods devoid of basic nutrients tends to promote an acidic environment—a pH<7.0 (typically <6.5). Examples of refined food to avoid are those that contain refined sugar, salt and oils.

Our bodies do not like to be in an acidic environment. An acidic environment is pro-inflammatory and most chronic illnesses, including cancers, are much more common in an acidic environment. Eating too much protein also promotes an acidic environment. What does our body do when the pH is too acidic (pH <6.0)? It releases calcium from the bones to buffer and raise the pH. A prolonged acidic pH will lead to osteopenia and osteoporosis.

How do you achieve a neutral pH? The number one way to maintain a neutral pH is to eat good food. Minerals are one of the most alkalinizing agents known. Most whole foods contain minerals at significantly higher amounts as compared to refined foods. In fact, most refined foods contain little or no minerals. Organic vegetables are some of the most alkalinizing foods. Unrefined salt is another example of an alkalinizing food substance. I have found it nearly impossible for many of my patients to raise their pH without the use of unrefined salt. For more information on salt, I refer the reader to my book, ***Salt Your Way to Health.***

Barbara, a 55-year-old auto worker was diagnosed with osteoporosis after having a bone mineral density test. "My doctor told me that if I didn't go on Fosomax®*, I would be crippled when I got older. That really scares me. I don't want to be all hunched over," she said. Barbara's BMD test showed that her T-score was -2.5 S.D., which gives her a diagnosis of osteoporosis. Barbara had tried Fosomax*®*, but could not tolerate the side effects. "It felt like it was burning my stomach and I am too young to take a medication for the rest of my life," she claimed. When I saw Barbara, I took a complete history, performed a physical exam and* ordered blood and urine tests. Barbara was found to have a very low morning salivary pH --6.0. She was also found to be low in many minerals including magnesium, potassium, boron, and zinc—all important minerals for building strong bones. Barbara was found to be very low in Vitamin D (15ng/ml) and Vitamin K (<0.2ng/ml). Barbara was placed on an organic diet that included lots of fruits and vegetables. She was told to avoid foods with refined sugar, flour, and salt. Barbara was instructed to ingest ½ tsp of unrefined sea salt (Celtic salt®) per day. Vitamin D (5,000I.U.) and Vitamin K (500µg) were also supplemented along with a good multivitamin and multimineral product. Within two weeks, Barbara's pH increased to 7.0. A repeat bone density one year later showed that her BMD test improved in all parameters. "I am so glad I did not take that drug. I feel so much better with the changes I have made. Even my friends are asking me what I am doing since I look so much better," she said.

Barbara's case is not unique. In fact, it occurs over and over in my practice. Osteoporosis can be effectively managed with a comprehensive plan that includes improving the diet and correcting vitamin and mineral imbalances. For proper bone health and strength, it is imperative to measure the pH and maintain a neutral pH. For more information on a healthy diet that is full of minerals, I refer the reader to my book, **_The Guide to Healthy Eating_**.

2. *AVOID OR MINIMIZE DAIRY*

I know many people (my mother?) may disagree with me on this section, but I encourage the readers to educate themselves and make their own decisions. The mainstream media has convinced us that the use of dairy products, and especially milk, can lead to strong bones and prevent osteoporosis. How wrong can they be?

A review of fracture rates of different countries found that the populations with the lowest calcium intake had the lowest fracture rate.[64] Another large review of 47 studies that looked at diary products and bone health found that 57% (27/47) found no relationship between dairy intake and bone mineralization in children and adolescents. Even the positive studies were only found to promote small or modest positive changes.[65] The Harvard Nurses Study of 77,761 women found the fracture rates were significantly higher for those who consumed three or more glasses of milk as compared to those that drank little or no milk.[66] A similar study of elderly men and women in Australia found that higher dairy product consumption was associated with an increased fracture risk.[67] Other studies have also found little correlation with dairy or calcium intake and bone gain or bone strength.[68]

We are one of the highest dairy consuming populations. We also have one of the highest rates of osteoporosis in the world. Dairy has never been shown to reduce the risk for developing osteoporosis and may actually increase the risk.

3. TAKE THE RIGHT FORM OF CALCIUM AND MAKE SURE YOU HAVE ADEQUATE AMOUNTS OF MINERALS

Calcium is the major mineral in bones. We do need adequate calcium from our diet and an adequate supply of calcium is essential to attain maximum bone mass. However, if we don't take the correct form and if we don't have the optimal amounts of other minerals, calcium will not find its way to the bones and may cause other problems.

Calcium citrate and lactate are the best absorbed forms of calcium. To ensure that calcium is absorbed from the GI tract, adequate Vitamin D must be present. Vitamin D levels can be ascertained from a serum blood test—25-OH D-3. My experience has clearly shown that low Vitamin D levels (<30ng/dl) are the norm in my patients. In fact, I believe low Vitamin D levels are occurring at epidemic levels. The reason Vitamin D levels have fallen in so many is due to people avoiding the sun and the overuse of sunscreen. Low Vitamin D levels have been associated with a host of illnesses including cancer of the breast, lung, and prostate as well as autoimmune disorders and osteoporosis. In the case of osteoporosis, with a Vitamin D deficiency, calcium cannot be absorbed from the gastrointestinal tract and it cannot be transported to the bones. In fact, the first test that should be performed in any evaluation of bone health should be a serum Vitamin D level.

Adequate levels of magnesium, boron, copper, zinc, silicon, and other minerals are important to ensure that the bones receive all the minerals that they need. Eating whole foods rich in minerals and supplementing with a good multi-mineral product can help.

Strontium is a trace element that helps strengthen bones. There are many studies showing strontium improving the strength and density of bones.[69][70][71][72][73] In fact, I have found the addition of 150mg of Strontium to an osteoporotic nutritional regimen an essential part of the treatment.

DHA, a fatty-acid component of fish oils has been shown in studies to maintain normal bone strength. Tocotrienols (a form of Vitamin E) are also important for bone health.

There are a whole host of nutrients that are beneficial for bone health. Nutrients, unlike the toxic bisphosphonate drugs, will not poison crucial enzymes or block important receptors. Nutrients will supply the body with the basic raw materials it needs to build and maintain healthy bones.

4. MAGNESIUM SUPPLEMENTATION AND OSTEOPOROSIS

Adequate levels of magnesium are necessary for the development and maintenance of bone health. Magnesium deficiency is one of the most common nutritional deficiencies that I see in my practice.

Magnesium has been shown to regulate calcium transport throughout the body. Studies have shown magnesium can prevent fractures and significantly increase bone density.[74] [75]

Taking calcium supplements when there is a magnesium deficiency can be problematic. When magnesium deficiency is present, calcium supplementation can alter the calcium/magnesium ratio. This can increase the risk of coagulation disorders.[76]

In order to maintain optimal bone strength, it is crucial to ensure adequate stores of magnesium. Ordering the correct test is important. A red blood cell magnesium test is an excellent way to assess magnesium levels. I do not recommend using the serum magnesium test. It is unreliable.

5. VITAMIN K

Vitamin K is necessary for the formation of the protein osteocalcin which helps attach calcium to the bones. Vitamin K supplementation was found to decrease the risk of:[77]

1. Hip fractures by 77%

2. Vertebral fractures by 60%

3. Non vertebral fractures by 81%

Vitamin K deficiency is very common in osteoporotic and osteopenic patients. 100-500µg of Vitamin K1 will be a positive addition to an osteoporotic regimen.

6. *VITAMIN B12 AND FOLIC ACID*

Deficiencies of Vitamin B12 and folic acid have been found to increase the risk of hip fractures.[78] Researchers found a significantly decreased risk of hip fractures in stroke patients treated with Vitamin B12 and folic acid versus subjects treated with a placebo. Pernicious anemia is a condition caused by a deficiency of Vitamin B12. Patients with pernicious anemia have been shown to have an elevated rate of bone fractures.

7: NATTOKINASE

Natto is fermented soy which contains the enzyme nattokinase. It is widely used in Japan. Researchers have shown an 80% reduction in bone density loss in postmenopausal women who consumed natto as compared to a group who did not consume natto.[79] This benefit increased the longer natto was ingested. Natto should be used by anyone suffering from osteoporosis. Natto is a good source of Vitamin K2. As previously mentioned, adequate Vitamin K levels are necessary for proper bone formation.

FINAL THOUGHTS: PUTTING IT ALL TOGETHER HOLISTICALLY

Eating a well balanced diet of whole foods, which helps the body maintain a neutral pH, will improve many conditions, including osteopenia and osteoporosis. Ensuring an adequate supply of minerals including calcium, magnesium, and other minerals is essential. Supplementing with strontium, Vitamin D, and Vitamin K will aid in bone strength. Daily exercise must also be part of any bone strengthening regimen. All of these components comprise a holistic way to treat osteoporosis, without the risk of any serious adverse effects. Bone and overall health will improve, but, most importantly, people will feel better on this regimen.

Osteoporosis drugs such as bisphosphonates should not be used, or at least used as a last resort. They have too many adverse effects and they are too disruptive to the body's normal physiology. Remember, *you can't poison a crucial enzyme or block an important receptor for the long-term and expect a good result.*

[1] NIH.gov accessed from: http://consensus.nih.gov/2000/2000Osteoporosis111html.htm. Accessed 8.11.06

[2] NIH. Gov accessed from: http://www.nof.org/osteoporosis/diseasefacts.htm

[3] U.S. Department of Health and Human Services. Bone health and osteoporosis: A report of the surgeon general. 10.14.04

[4] FP News. July 1, 2006

[5] IBID. U.S. Department of Health and Human Services. Bone health and osteoporosis: A report of the surgeon general.

[6] National Osteoporosis Foundation. Accessed from: nof.org 8.12.06

[7] IBID. U.S. Department of Health and Human Services. 10.14.04

[8] J. of Clin. Endocr. and Metab. July 2006;91(7). 2600-2604

[9] National Osteoporosis Foundation. Accessed from: nof.org 8.12.06

[10] Genant, H. Interim report and recommendations ofhte WHO Task-Force for Osteoporosis. Osteoporosis International. 1999;19:259-264

[11] Samson, G. The Myth of Osteoporosis. MCD Century publications. 2003

[12] WHO

[13] Samson, G. IBID. 2003.

[14] NIH.gov accessed from: http://consensus.nih.gov/2000/2000Osteoporosis111html.htm. Accessed 8.11.06

[15] Green, C.J., Et al. Bone mineral testing: Does the evidence support its selective use in well women? British Columbia Office of Health TECHNOLOGY Assessment. Dec. 1997.

[16] Helfand, M as quoted in Homemaker's 1998. Oct. 1998;57-70

[17] Kazanjian, A. International J. of Technology Assessment in Health Care 1999. 15:679-685

[18] JAMA 7/17/02. Vol. 288, No. 3

[19] Cummings, SR. Risk factors for hip fracture in white women. Study of osteoporotic fractures research group. N. Eng. J. Med. 1995;332:767-773

[20] Goddard, D. The epidemiology of osteoporosis. Post Graduate Medicine. Vol. 104. No. 4. Oct. 1998

[21] FP News. 01/05

[22] Hart, JP. Electrochemical detection of depressed circulating levels of Vitamin K1 in osteoporosis. J.Clin. Endocrin. Metabl. 1985;60:1268-69

[23] Soontrapa, S. J. Med. Assoc. Thail. 2005. Oct;88 Supple. 5:s29-32

[24] Hart, JT. Circulating Vitamin K levels in fractured neck of femur. Lancet. 1984;2:283

[25] Caraballo, PJ. Arch. Int. Med. 1999. Aug9-23;159(15):1750-6

[26] Wright, J. In Dr. Jonathan V. Wright's Nutrition and Healing Newsletter. Vol. 7. Issue 7. July 2000.

[27] National Institute of Health Consensus Development Conference Statement. Osteoporosis prevention, diagnosis and therapy. 2000. Accessed from: http//consensus.nih.gov/2000/2000osteoporosis111html.htm

[28] IBID. National Institute of Health Consensus Development Conference Statement. 2000

[29] McGrother, CW. Evaluation of a hip fracture risk score for assessing elderly women: The Melton Osteoporotic Fracture Study. Osteoporosis International 2002;13:89-96

[30] Fasano, A. Prevalence of celiac disease in at-risk and not-at-risk groups in the U.S. A large mulitcenter study. Archives of Int. Med. 2003;163:286-292

[31] The effects of 1-year gluten withdrawal on bone mass, bone metabolism and nutritional status in newly-diagnosed adult celiac disease patients. Alimentary Pharm. and Therap. 2000. Jan:14(I):35-43

[32] Feskaich, D. Milk, dietary calcium, and bone fractures in women; a 12 year prospective study. Am. J. of Public Health. 1997;87:992-7

[33] Lloyd, T. Lifestyle factors and the development of bone mass and bone strength in young women. J. Pediatr. 2004; Jun;144(6):776-82

[34] Lanou, A.J. Calcium, diary products, and bone health in children and young adults: a reevaluation of the evidence. Pediatrics. 2005. Mar;115(3):736-43

[35] Weinsier, R. Dairy foods and bone health: examination of the evidence. Am. J. Clin. Nutr. 2000. Sept. 72(3):681-9

[36] Fraser, Ian. Estrogens and progestogens. Clin. Practice. London, Eng. Curchiill, Livingston. 1998;275-276. p. 658

[37] Clinical pharmacology online.

[38] J. Clin. Endocrin. Metab. 2001. Jun;86(6):2437-45

[39] Gertz, BJ. Clinical pharmacology of alendronate sodium. Osteoporos. Int. 1993;3 Suppl. 3:S13-6.

[40] From Pharmacy Times. http://www.pharmacytimes.com/article.cfm?ID=2534

[41] Sama, AA. High-dose alendronate uncouples osteoclasts and osteoblasts function: a study in rat spine pseudarthrosis model. Clin Orthop. Relat. Res. 2004 Aug;(425):135-42

[42] Huang, RC. Spine. 2005. Von. 15;30(22):2516-22

[43] Lehman, RA. The effect of alendronate sodium n spinal fusion: a rabbit mode. Spine J. 2004. Jan-Feb;4(1):36-43

[44] Black, DM. Fracture intervention trial research group. Randomized trial of effect of alendronate on risk of fracture in women with existing vertebral fractures. Lancet. 1996;348:1535-1541

[45] Sanson, G. IBID.

[46] Black, Dm> Randomized trial of effect of alendronate on risk of fracture in women with existing vertebral fractures. Lancet. 1996;348:1535-41

[47] Cummings, S.R. Effect of alendronate on risk of fracture in women with low bone density but without vertebral fractures. JAMA. 1998;280(24):1077-82

[48] Braun, E. Bisphosphonates: Case report of nonsurgical periodontal therapy and osteochemonecrosis. The Int. J. of Periodontics and Restorative Dentistry. Vol. 26, No. 4. 2006

[49] J. Oral Maxillofac. Implants. 1995;10:74-8

[50] J. Oral. Maxillofac. Surg. 2004;62:527-34

[51] J. Oral. Maxillofac. Surg. 2005;63:682-9

[52] Clin. Implant. Dent. Relat. Res. 2003;5;269-72

[53] J. Periodontol. 2002;73:813-22

[54] Endo, Y. Calcif. Tissue. Int. 1993. Mar;52(3):248-54

[55] Shimshi, M. Bisphosphonates induce inflammation and rupture of atherosclerotic plaques in apoliporteitn-E nul mice. Biochem. Biophys. Res. Commun. 2005. Mar. 18;328(3):790-3

[56] Richards, Byron. Fight for Your Heath. Truth in Wellness Books. 2006.

[57] J. Rheumatology. 2004. Apr. 31(4):829-30

[58] Invest. Clin. 2002. Mar;43(1):49-52

[59] Gastroenterol. Clin. Biol. 2002. Feb;26(2):179-80

[60] J. Am. Acad. Dermatol. 2003. J un;48(6):945-6

[61] CMAF. 2002. Jan8;166(1)86-7

[62] National Osteoporosis Foundation. www.nof.org

[63] Sanson, G. IBID. pg. 72

[64] Abelow, BJ. Cross-cultural association between dietary animal protein and hip fracture: a hypothesis. Calif. Tissue. Int. 1992;50:14-8

[65] Lanou, AF. Calcium, dairy products, and bone health in children and young adults.: a reevaluation of the evidence. Pediatrics. 2005. Mar;115(3):736-43

[66] Feskanich, D. Milk, dietary calcium, and bone fractures in women: a 12-year prospective study. Am. J. Pub. Health. 1997;87:992-7

[67] Cumming, RG. Case-control study of risk factors for hip fractures in the elderly. Am. J. Epidemiol. 1994;139:493-503

[68] Lloyd, T. Lifestyle factors and the development of bone mass and bone strength in young women. J. Pediatr. 2004.Jun;144(6):776-82

[69] McCaslin, FE. The effect of strontium lactate in the treatment of osteoporosis. Proc. Staff. Meetings. Mayo Clin. 1959, 34:329-334

[70] Marie, P.J. Short-term effects of fluoride and strontium on bone formation and resorption in the mouse. Metab. 1986, 35:547-551

[71] Meunier, P.J., Slosman, D.O., Delmas, P.D., Sebert, J.L., Brandi, M.L., Albanese, C., Lorenc, R., Pors-Nielsen, S., De Vernejoul, M.C., Roces, A., Reginster J.Y. Strontium ranelate: dose-dependent effects in established postmenopausal vertebral osteoporosis—a 2-year randomized placebo controlled trial. J Clin Endocrinol Metab, May 2002; 87(5):2060-6.

[72] Meunier, P.J., Roux, C., Seeman, E., Ortolani, S., Badurski, J.E., Spector, T.D., Cannata, J., Balogh, A., Lemmel, E.M., Pors-Nielsen, S., Rizzoli R., Genant, H.K., Reginster J.Y. The effects of strontium ranelate on the risk of vertebral fracture in women with postmenopausal osteoporosis, N Engl J Med, 2004, Jan 29;350(5):459-68.

[73] Ortolani S, Vai S. Strontium ranelate: An increased bone quality leading to vertebral antifracture efficacy at all stages. Bone. 2006 Jan 30;38(2S1):19-22

[74] Sojka, J. Nutr. Rev. 1995. Mar;53(3):71-4

[75] Abraham, G. J. Reprod. Med. 1990. May;35(5):503-7

[76] Seelig, M. J. Am. Coll. Nutr. 1993. Aug;12(4):442-58

[77] Cockayne, S. Vitamin K and the prevention of fractures. Arch. Intern. Med. 2006;166:1256-61

[78] Sato, Y. Effect of folate and methylcobalamin on hip fractures in patients with stroke. JAMA. 2005;293:1082-3

[79] Ikeda,Y. Intake of fermented soybeans, natto, is associated with reduced bone loss in postmenopausal women: Japanese population-based osteoporosis study. J. Nutr. 2006;136(5): 1323-8

Chapter 6

Antacid Drugs

INTRODUCTION

Stomach acid must be bad for you. That is the message from all of the ads that you see on television and in the magazines. The connotation is clear: if you have gastric (stomach) pain or esophagus pain, too much stomach acid must be the culprit and stomach acid needs to be limited.

Big Pharma began to promote the idea that stomach acid is bad for you shortly after they developed a plethora of pills to reduce the production of stomach acid. If you walk into your local pharmacy or grocery store, the antacid section in these stores is enormous. There are shelves and shelves of antacid medications containing:

1. Over-the-counter medications that neutralize stomach acid such as Alka Seltzer®, Mylanta®, or Maalox®.

2. The older medications (H-2 blockers) that decrease acid production such as Tagamet®, Axid®, Zantac®, or Pepcid®.

3. The newest and most effective medications which inhibit acid production (proton pump inhibitors) such as Nexium®, Aciphex®, Prevacid®, Protonix®, Zegerid® and Prilosec®.

As can be seen from the previous page, there are a wide range of choices to neutralize, lower, or block your body's production of stomach acid.

This chapter will show you that you do need adequate amounts of stomach acid. A deficiency of stomach acid results in multiple digestive problems, vitamin and mineral deficiencies, and a downward spiral in your health.

All health begins and ends in the gastrointestinal tract. If we cannot properly digest and absorb nutrients from our food, we set the stage for an imbalanced immune system and the onset and progression of chronic illness.

I have worked closely with my patients over the last 17 years to evaluate and treat a multitude of digestive complaints. Out of hundreds, if not thousands of patients tested, I have only found one patient who produces excess stomach acid. In fact, when I measure stomach acid levels--directly via a Heidelberg Test or indirectly by a comprehensive stool digestive analysis--one thing has been clear; lowered stomach acid production is a common condition in many of those suffering from digestive complaints. That might seem like a contradiction; how can lowered stomach acid produce many of the complaints that antacid medications seem to help? This chapter will explain the answer to this question and why it is important to ensure adequate stomach acid levels, particularly as you age. I will also show how the use of natural supplements can help with stomach acid problems. Finally, this chapter will explain why antacid medications should be used only as a last resort.

HOW DOES THE STOMACH DIGEST FOOD?

Stomach acid (hydrochloric acid—HCL) is secreted by specialized cells in the stomach called parietal cells. Parietal cells respond to the hormone gastrin.

When food enters the stomach, the pH (a measure of acidity) rises which signals the gastric cells to release gastrin. Gastrin is the messenger hormone to the parietal cells giving the command to release hydrochloric acid resulting in a lowered pH which facilitates the digestion of food.

The stomach maintains an acidic condition at rest by secreting small amounts of hydrochloric acid to maintain a pH of 1-3. A special lining is present in the stomach to protect itself from this highly acidic environment. In fact, the stomach was designed to function optimally at this very acidic pH.

Everything is in balance if the stomach is properly maintaining an acidic pH by producing optimal amounts of hydrochloric acid in order to do its job--digest food. When there is an imbalance in the pH, digestive problems develop.

CAN THE STOMACH PRODUCE TOO MUCH HYDROCHLORIC ACID?

Yes.   Hypergastrinemia is an uncommon condition whereby the gastric cells of the stomach secrete large amounts of gastrin. The excess gastrin can result in an excess of hydrochloric acid being secreted. Certain tumors and genetic conditions can predispose one to a hypergastrinemic situation.

The most potent inhibitor of gastrin production is the amount of hydrochloric acid in the stomach.[1] When there is an adequate amount of hydrochloric acid in the stomach, a negative feedback loop ensues which sends the signal to lower gastrin levels. Conversely, if the pH is too high, gastrin levels will increase in order to stimulate the production of hydrochloric acid. The proton pump inhibitors so commonly prescribed today--including Nexium®and Prilosec®--shut off all hydrochloric acid production. This leads to elevated gastrin levels--known as hypergastrinemia-- being secreted in the stomach. More about proton pump inhibitors will follow.

Hypergastrinemia has been associated with gastric cancer and non-gastric cancers. Colon cancer has been found to be associated with high gastrin levels.[2] In animals, elevated gastrin levels have been associated with cancers of the gastrointestinal tract.[3]

H. pylori is a pathogenic bacteria found in the stomach. Infection with H. pylori is associated with significant gastrointestinal disease as well as causing excess gastrin to be released.[4] However, H. pylori infection is often not associated with too much stomach acid; in fact, it is often associated with too little stomach acid.

CAN THE STOMACH PRODUCE TOO LITTLE HYDROCHLORIC ACID?

Yes. Achlorhydria is a condition whereby too little hydrochloric acid is produced in the stomach and the pH of the stomach cannot fall to less than 4.0. Remember, normal pH in the stomach is 1-3.

As previously mentioned, a higher pH (>4.0) will stimulate the gastrin cells to increase their production of gastrin. Higher gastrin levels are the stomach's response to achlorhydria. Elevated gastrin levels may not be a good thing as these elevated levels have been shown to increase the risk of developing gastric and colon cancers.

Achlorhydria can be caused by many conditions—see Table 1. Of particular interest is the association of low stomach acid with H. pylori infection and long-term use of proton pump inhibitors. More about this topic later. The long term use of proton pump inhibitors such as Nexium® and Prilosec® can result in an irreversible achlorhydric state. What are the effects of using proton pump inhibitors for the long-term? No one knows. However, common sense would suggest that it is not a good idea to inhibit acid production for the long term. In fact, it is best to use these drugs only for a short course—less than four weeks. For the long term, proton pump inhibitors will inevitably lead to serious adverse effects. More about proton pump inhibitors will be discussed later in this chapter. Further information on the benefits of maintaining adequate stomach acid levels can be found in **_Why Stomach Acid Is Good For You_** by Jonathan Wright, M.D.

Table 1: Conditions Which May Cause Achlorhydria

1. Pernicious anemia
2. Autoimmune thyroid disease
3. H. pylori infection
4. Mucolipidosis type IV
5. Long-term treatment with proton pump inhibitors

Achlorhydria can be caused by pernicious anemia. Pernicious anemia is an autoimmune condition of the stomach. It causes an elevated stomach pH and raises gastrin levels. Vitamin B-12 deficiency and gastric cancers are much more common in pernicious anemia.

WHAT ARE THE EIGHT CONSEQUENCES OF LOW STOMACH ACID?

1. VITAMIN B-12 DEFICIENCY

As previously mentioned, low stomach acid is associated with an increase in gastric cancer, colon cancer, H. pylori infection and pernicious anemia. In addition, proper amounts of hydrochloric acid in the stomach are necessary for vitamin and mineral absorption.

Vitamin B-12 deficiency is rampant in our modern society. B-12 deficiency is associated with a host of ailments including fatigue[5], fibromyalgia, hip fractures[6], chronic fatigue, glossitis (swollen tongue), and anemia[7]. In addition, B-12 deficiency has been associated with many neurological disorders.[8] Depression, confusion, dementia, and difficulty in maintaining balance (especially with the elderly) are also common with Vitamin B-12 deficiency.[9] All patients with achlorhydria, including those on proton pump inhibitors (e.g., Nexium® and Prilosec®), need to have their Vitamin B-12 levels evaluated and treated with Vitamin B-12 injections when indicated. Oral preparations of Vitamin B-12 will not be absorbed well when there is suboptimal production of stomach acid. My clinical experience has been clear; almost all patients on antacid drugs are deficient in Vitamin B-12. Injectable forms of Vitamin B12 (hydroxyl or methyl B12) have proven very successful. For most people, I recommend using injectable Vitamin B12 when supplementing with Vitamin B12. My clinical experience has clearly shown that oral, nasal, and sublingual forms of Vitamin B12 are not as effective as injectable Vitamin B12.

2. BACTERIAL OVERGROWTH OF THE STOMACH

Achlorhydria is also associated with bacterial overgrowth of the stomach. One of the main reasons the stomach produces so much acid is to kill the bacteria and other pathogenic organisms in our food. Adequate stomach acid production will not allow toxic bacteria to colonize our gastrointestinal tract. If the pH of the stomach is too high, the anti-bacterial activity of hydrochloric acid is lost. Many articles have been written about gastrointestinal bacterial overgrowth due to the use of antacid drugs. Bacterial overgrowth is common in many gastrointestinal disorders including irritable bowel syndrome, Crohn's disease, and ulcerative colitis.

3. H. PYLORI INFECTION

H. pylori infection occurs in approximately 20% of persons younger than 40 years and 50% of those over 60 years. How can a pathogenic bacterium be affecting over 50% of those over 60 years old? Many factors contribute to this, including a poor diet consisting of refined sugar, trans fats, and refined salt. However, the number one factor that I see in my practice predisposing to H. pylori is achlorhydria or low stomach acid.

If the pH of the stomach is in a normal range (pH 1-3), my experience has shown that H. pylori infections are rare. When there is inadequate production of hydrochloric acid, H. pylori infections are much more common. Conventional treatment for H. pylori involves using a short-term therapy of proton pump inhibitors and antibiotics. This short-term therapy is effective for eradicating H.pylori.

However, I have witnessed a high rate of recurrence of H. pylori when long-term (>1 month) acid suppression with a proton pump inhibitor is used. If a normal pH is maintained in the stomach (i.e., acidic), my experience has been clear; H. pylori infection is rare. More information about H. pylori and a natural way to treat H. pylori, without blocking acid production, can be found on later in this chapter.

Ruth, 72-years-old, was complaining of a burning feeling in her stomach. "My stomach just does not feel right. I am feeling bloated and it hurts much of the time," she said. Ruth was treated with Nexium®, a proton-pump inhibitor. Although some of her burning pain was helped with Nexium®, she still had discomfort. "I know my stomach is not right. I can't eat anything without some pain," she said. Ruth tested positive for H. pylori. Ruth was prescribed a course of antibiotics to treat H. pylori. However, she did not want to take the antibiotics. "I have such bowel problems with antibiotics," she said. When Ruth called her son (the holistic medical doctor), he told her that he had successfully treated many people with H. pylori infections without the use of antacids or antibiotics. In fact, her son told her that antibiotics and antacids should only be used if the herbal therapies fail. Ruth was treated with oregano oil (50mg three times per day), mastic (500 mg/day), acidophilus powder (1/2tsp two times per day) and aloe vera gel (two tbsp three times per day). She was also instructed to stop Nexium®. Within three days, all of her symptoms improved. "It felt so wonderful to feel normal again. I was thrilled I did not have to take an antibiotic as they always cause me more problems," she said.

Ruth is my mother. Having your mother ill is not a good thing. My mother has had two further recurrences of H. pylori infections and both were successfully treated with the above regimen.

4. C. DIFFICILE INFECTION AND ACID-BLOCKING MEDICATIONS

C. difficile is a bacterium that can infect the colon and cause severe diarrhea. It causes over three million cases of diarrhea and colitis per year in the United States. In fact, more than 1% of all U.S. hospitalized patients are infected with C. difficile.[10] C. difficile infections used to be primarily seen in hospitalized patients on I.V. antibiotics. Antibiotics will kill normal intestinal flora as well as pathogenic bacteria. If enough of the normal flora is killed off, C. difficile bacteria can overgrow and cause problems. Approximately 3% of patients with C. difficile colitis develop fulminant colitis which can be fatal. Approximately 20% of people infected with C. difficile will have repeated bouts of the illness and approximately 1-4% die from the illness.[11] [12] Before the introduction of acid blocking medications, C. difficile was rarely seen in the outpatient setting. In the past, it was primarily seen in hospitalized patients in the intensive care unit who were under tremendous stress and treated with powerful antibiotics. C. difficile infections are costly; in 2002, over $1.6 billion was spent on patients hospitalized for C. difficile infections.[13] That figure only includes hospitalized costs; when you factor in out-patient costs, the estimates would markedly increase.

However, since the introduction of powerful antacid medications, there has been a dramatic upward trend of C. difficile infections. The incidence of C. difficile has been increasing from less than 1 case per 100,000 in 1994 to over 22 per 100,000 in 2004. Estimates are that from 225,000 to 500,000 new cases of C. difficile infections are occurring annually.[14] One study found that there was a 290% increase in C. difficile in people that take proton pump inhibitors such as Nexium®.[15] The same study found a 200% increase in C. difficile infection in those taking H-2 blockers such as Zantac®, Pepcid® or Axid®.

The reason we are seeing such a dramatic increase in C. difficile infections is clear; it is due to the overuse of powerful antacid medications. Acid blockers will change the pH of the stomach. The highly acidic environment of the stomach not only serves the purpose of digesting food and absorbing minerals, it also helps to kill bacteria, yeast, and parasites that we may ingest. On the other hand, blocking this acidic environment will tend to promote abnormal growth of bacteria, yeast, and parasites in the gastrointestinal tract. A low stomach acid environment ultimately leads to a whole host of gastrointestinal problems including C. difficile infections.

5. *YEAST AND CANDIDA OVERGROWTH AND LOW STOMACH ACID*

My clinical experience has shown that yeast overgrowth of the bowel is very common when there is a low amount of stomach acid present. As previously mentioned, an adequate stomach pH is needed to not only digest food, but to kill ingested yeast and other microorganisms. Furthermore, I have found it extremely difficult to effectively treat yeast (or Candida) overgrowth when a patient is taking an antacid medication.

6. INADEQUATE PROTEIN INTAKE AND LOW STOMACH ACID

Low stomach acid is also associated with a poor digestion of protein. This will lead to a low protein state in the body. Pepsinogen A, an enzyme that helps digest protein, is markedly low in achlorhydria.[16] [17] [18] Adequate protein provides the body with the necessary ingredients to promote structural integrity. My clinical experience has shown that low protein states are associated with many degenerative disorders including fibromyalgia, chronic fatigue syndrome, cancer, and arthritic disorders. It is very difficult for the body to heal injured tissue when there is inadequate protein absorbed from the diet.

7. MINERAL DEFICIENCIES AND LOW STOMACH ACID

Mineral deficiencies are common with inadequate stomach acid. Iron[19], zinc, copper, and calcium are common deficiencies observed in achlorhydria. In fact, I have found it nearly impossible to balance a patient's mineral status if there is inadequate stomach acid present.

8. LOW STOMACH ACID AND HYPOTHYROIDISM

For those taking thyroid hormone, impaired stomach acid production has been found to decrease the absorption of thyroid hormone by approximately 25%.[20] The implications of this study are tremendous. Estimates are that from 10-40% of the adult population in the U.S. has a thyroid illness. I have no doubt that the tremendous amount of thyroid illnesses found in the U.S. is being driven, in part, by the overuse of antacid medications. If you are taking an acid-blocking drug and you are concurrently on thyroid medication, you may need to increase your thyroid dose by 25% to compensate.

Antacid drugs, by lowering the absorption of protein, can also cause a hypothyroid condition. If the body is not able to get the proper nutrition it needs, it will slow the metabolism down. Hypothyroidism is associated with a lowered metabolism. I have seen many patients with all of the clinical features of hypothyroidism dramatically improve their condition when their body is supplied with the correct nutrients such as adequate amounts of protein.

WHAT IS HEARTBURN?

Who hasn't had an episode of heartburn? Most of us have had at least one episode of heartburn after eating greasy food. When you take an antacid while you are having heartburn, the pain immediately dissipates. Wouldn't that mean that the pain is caused by too much acid?

The answers to these questions seem simple. The ads from Big Pharma would make it seem that heartburn is the result of too much acid being produced in the stomach. These ads imply that shutting down acid production is all that is needed to treat/prevent heartburn. As we previously discussed, ensuring a low stomach acid production may not be in your best interest as it has been shown to cause cancer and vitamin deficiencies, as well as bacterial, yeast, and parasitic overgrowth. In addition low stomach acid has been associated with serious gastrointestinal disorders such as colitis and other serious health issues.

Maybe we should look at the pain from heartburn as a symptom of an underlying health issue. Perhaps it is the body's way of informing you of a problem in your stomach, esophagus, or wherever the pain is originating from.

Heartburn pain can be a sign that the lower esophageal sphincter is not working. The lower esophageal sphincter is designed to keep the acidic stomach contents from regurgitating up the esophagus where it can burn the esophageal tissue. There are many reasons why the lower esophageal sphincter does not work correctly. The number one reason is too much abdominal fat. Too much abdominal fat will put pressure on the stomach and may weaken the sphincter over time. A hiatal hernia can also cause problems with the sphincter.

Many times lowering the pH of the stomach will actually make the lower esophageal sphincter work much better.

Ellis, age 64, had been treated with Zantac® and Prilosec® (medications to block stomach acid production) for five years. He complained of constant heartburn after he ate. "It feels like a fire coming up my chest right after I am done eating," he said. Ellis got some relief from Zantac, but still suffered. He said, "When I started the medication, I felt much better, but over time it wasn't working as well. Sometimes I have to stop my meals in the middle because the pain is too much." Ellis was found to have reflux esophagitis by a gastrointestinal doctor. His lower esophageal sphincter was not doing its job of keeping the stomach contents out of the esophagus. When I saw Ellis, I ordered a Heidelberg test which showed that the pH in his stomach was too high from inadequate hydrochloric acid production. I instructed him to stop the acid-blocking medications and to take hydrochloric acid pills with his meals--six grains with each meal. Ellis experienced immediate relief. "It was a miracle. All my pain was gone and stayed gone if I took the pills. If I forgot them, it returned," he said. Ellis went to his gastrointestinal doctor and told him how much better he was doing. The doctor did not believe it. He told him to stop the hydrochloric acid pills and go back on the acid -blocking pills. "I told him how much better I was doing and he did not care. He kept telling me I was producing too much stomach acid. When I asked him if he measured the stomach acid, he said he did not have to," Ellis said. Ellis decided to continue with the hydrochloric acid pills. A follow-up scope by the gastrointestinal doctor showed no irritation in his esophagus even though he was taking the hydrochloric acid.

Ellis is my father. He used to enjoy telling his friends who were taking the expensive antacid medications that he was taking stomach acid pills to help his digestion.

I suggest you seek care with a holistic practitioner skilled in the use of natural items before trying hydrochloric acid pills on your own. If you have any burning in your stomach or chest while taking the pills, stop and seek medical attention. A Heidelberg test can measure the stomach acid pH. This test can be a good guide on whether you need supplementation with hydrochloric acid.

The use of antacids to treat heartburn does not treat the underlying cause of the illness. The pain due to reflux is not the result of an 'antacid deficiency'. In most cases it is not due to an excessive production of stomach acid. My experience has shown that reflux pain can be due to many different causes including obesity, inadequate stomach acid production, and infection. More about reflux can be found in the gastroesophageal reflux section found later in this chapter. In order to successfully treat any condition including heartburn, the underlying cause of the pain must be searched for. Once the underlying cause of the illness is identified, then you can formulate a comprehensive and effective long-term treatment plan.

GASTRITIS

The stomach has special cells in it--mucous cells--that secrete mucus which helps protect the stomach lining from the acidic environment.   When there is inadequate mucous production, hydrochloric acid can damage the stomach lining. An ulcer (hole) in the stomach is a common problem when there is inadequate mucous production. When hydrochloric acid contacts an ulcer, it is painful. Patients will report a burning pain in the pit of the stomach in the case of a stomach ulcer. In this case, the short-term (1-4 weeks) use of a proton pump inhibitor (e.g., Nexium or Prilosec) to limit acid production is an appropriate therapy. Once the ulcer is healed, the acid blockade can be removed. Licorice root is a very effective natural therapy that helps coat the stomach lining. If the damage to the mucosa is not severe, I have found licorice root a very effective treatment for gastritis, without the need for an antacid medication. Damage to the lining of the stomach coupled with a low stomach acid production can predispose one to bacterial infections such as H. pylori.

H. PYLORI INFECTIONS

H. pylori is a spiral-shaped bacterium that is found in the gastric mucosa or adherent to the epithelial lining of the stomach. Approximately two-thirds of the world's population is infected with H. pylori.[21] H. pylori infections are thought to cause up to 80% of gastric ulcers and 90% of duodenal ulcers.[22] H. pylori can be diagnosed either by a blood test, biopsy, or a breath test.

The conventional method for treating H. pylori infections involves using a combination of antibiotics and acid blockers. There are currently eight regimens of antibiotics/acid blocker combinations that are FDA-approved to treat H. pylori. These treatments are effective at eradicating H. pylori.

However, H. pylori has not infected two-thirds of the world's population due to a deficiency of acid blocking medications and antibiotics. Common sense would suggest that you should correct the underlying conditions that lead to the development of H. pylori. Treating the underlying conditions will help the body's own defense mechanisms eradicate H. pylori without the use of acid-blocking drugs. This results in an improved immune system and a much lower chance of recurrence.

How can H. pylori be infecting over two-thirds of the world's population? I believe that poor diets coupled with the increasing exposure to toxins in our environment are the primary reasons H. pylori infection has become so rampant. A poor diet will not only lead to a suboptimal immune system, it decreases the ability of the body to fight infections such as H. pylori.

What is a poor diet? It is a diet high in refined foods, especially refined sugars. Refined food provides no nutrition for our bodies. In fact, our bodies have to use their own store of nutrients to try and digest these lifeless foods. The long-term intake of refined foods will lead to a long-term depletion of various vitamins, minerals and enzymes that ultimately causes a downward spiral in health. H. pylori infection is one consequence of a poor diet.

I have consistently observed dramatic improvements in my patients who suffer from H. pylori when they eliminate refined sugar from their diet. Refined sugar feeds abnormal bacterium such as H. pylori. It is much more difficult to eliminate H. pylori if one continues to ingest refined sugars and other lifeless foods. My experience has also shown that refined salt exacerbates a H. pylori infection. Refined salt, like all refined food needs to be avoided. More information on how to avoid refined foods can be found in **_The Guide to Healthy Eating_** and **_Salt Your Way to Health._**

HOW TO TREAT H. PYLORI HOLISTICALLY

Part of any successful H. pylori treatment has to encompass dietary changes. As previously mentioned, eliminating refined foods is one of the best remedies for eradicating H. pylori. Maintaining a normal pH in the stomach (an acidic pH) is essential to help the body eradicate H. pylori.

Whenever H. pylori is diagnosed or suspected, the pH of the stomach should be measured initially. If the pH of the stomach is too high, a trial of hydrochloric acid supplementation is indicated. One to ten grains (60-600mg) of hydrochloric acid with meals will often improve the situation. If one experiences excess burning with hydrochloric acid supplementation, it should not be taken. If there is an ulceration of the gastric lining, hydrochloric acid supplementation should not be given until the ulceration is healed.

In addition to ensuring an adequate pH of the stomach, I recommend taking the herbal supplement mastic. Mastic is produced by a perennial shrub native to the Mediterranean region. Mastic resin seeps from the bark of the plant and contains the active ingredients that are effective for eradicating H. pylori. Mastic has been shown to be effective at treating duodenal ulcers in a double blind controlled trial.[23] Over 90% of duodenal ulcers have been associated with H. pylori infections.[24] The New England Journal of Medicine reported the ability of mastic to kill H. pylori bacteria in 1998.[25] The side effects from mastic are few; occasionally an upset stomach will occur. Mastic should be the first item used in any H. pylori infection. It is far less expensive and causes much fewer adverse effects than the FDA-approved Big Pharma recommended regimen of antibiotics and acid-blockers.

My experience has shown that mastic also has other positive effects such as preventing cavities and inhibiting candida overgrowth. Mastic can be taken in tablet form or chewed as gum. An effective dose of mastic is 500mg three times per day, taken without food.

In addition, oregano oil has proved to be a wonderful agent at helping the body overcome H. pylori. My experience has shown that 50mg of oregano oil (sustained release works the best) three times per day, with meals, has consistently shown positive effects in eradicating H. pylori.

Finally, adding in a source of acidiphillous bacteria has proven helpful in the treatment of H. Pylori bacteria.

The commonly prescribed antibiotic regimens for H. pylori are also effective for eradicating the illness. However, the antibiotics not only kill the bad bacteria (H. pylori), but will also harm the good intestinal bacteria such as L. acidophilus.

In the case of H. pylori infection, I feel the natural therapy as outlined above is a better initial course of treatment as compared to Big Pharma's patented antibiotic/antacid regimen. My clinical experience has proven it to be a very effective treatment regimen. The cost of the herbal therapy is much less expensive than the commonly prescribed antibiotic regimen: Approximately $25 for the herbal approach versus $333.00 (14-day course) for the prescription antibiotic approach.

If the above herbal approach does not provide complete relieve, adding in zinc and L-carnosine along with cranberry juice can be the answer. Numerous studies have shown that a combination of zinc and the naturally occurring amino acid L-carnosine can effectively treat stomach ulcers and have an inhibitory effect on H. pylori.[26] [27] [28] Cranberry has also been found to be effective at inhibiting the growth of H. pylori.[29] I recommend regular consumption of pure cranberry juice if you suffer from H. pylori infections.

GASTROESOPHAGEAL REFLUX DISEASE—GERD

Burning pain that goes up the chest is frequently diagnosed as gastroesophageal reflux disease or GERD. The esophagus is the muscular tube that begins in the back of the throat and ends at the upper part of the stomach. The esophagus is lined with epithelial cells and is not designed to be in contact with hydrochloric acid. It does not have the protective coating and the protective cells that the stomach has. Even if a small amount of stomach acid contacts the esophagus, it can damage the esophageal epithelial cells which results in pain and GERD.

GERD can be a serious condition. Long time exposure of the esophagus to hydrochloric acid can change the cells lining the esophagus resulting in a pre-cancerous condition known as Barrett's esophagus. The risk of esophageal cancer increases by 30-50 times if Barrett's esophagus is present.

Over seven million people in the United States are affected by GERD.[30] The lower esophageal sphincter (LES) is a muscular ring at the bottom of the esophagus that will open to let food into the stomach and close after the food has passed. GERD occurs when the LES does not close properly and the stomach contents can leak back into the esophagus.

What causes GERD? Most times, there is not one single cause. Table 2 gives some of the most common causes of GERD.

TABLE 2: CAUSES OF GERD
1. Alcohol use
2. Obesity
3. Pregnancy
4. Smoking

When I have measured hydrochloric acid levels with a Heidelberg Test (or indirectly via a comprehensive stool digestive analysis) in patients who are having GERD, over 90% of time I have found low hydrochloric acid levels. It is extremely rare to find elevated or even normal HCL production in these patients. The next time you are told to take an acid blocker for GERD or other stomach issues, ask to have your gastric pH checked.

Certain foods can be associated with GERD. These include spicy foods, citrus foods, chocolate, caffeine, and fried foods. Conventional medicine treats GERD by suggesting dietary changes including eliminating alcohol and smoking, as well as eliminating foods that tend to cause GERD symptoms. If those changes fail, prescriptions for acid-blockers will be given. Since they have so many side effects, acid blocking medications should be used only as a last resort. However, there are safe and effective natural therapies to treat GERD.

CHILDREN AND GERD

Many parents are treating their newborn children with acid-blocking medications. Doctors are all too quick to diagnose reflux in a newborn that spits up. Once the diagnosis is made, the parents are oftentimes encouraged to place their newborn on an antacid medication. There are many steps to take before giving your newborn baby an acid-blocking medication. Medications should be the absolute last step. Very few children require an acid blocking medication.

Simple steps like decreasing the amount of food at one sitting and changing the formula should be tried first. Diagnosing and eliminating food allergies is a very important step for a child who is suffering from spitting up. An acupressure technique, NAET, has proven very effective at helping a child overcome a food allergy. For more information on NAET, please look at www.naet.com.

FOUR STEPS TO TREAT GERD HOLISTICALLY

1. *LOSE WEIGHT AND EAT LESS*

My experience has shown that eliminating or decreasing alcohol use and cigarette smoking significantly improves GERD symptoms. Both alcohol and cigarettes decrease the effectiveness of the lower esophageal sphincter (LES). When the LES becomes weak, it will allow stomach acid to leak into the esophagus.

The two main causes of GERD are obesity and overeating. Obesity is associated with excess weight around the abdomen. This excess fat pad will push the stomach upwards. As the stomach is pushed upwards, it will decrease the effectiveness of the LES and can lead to GERD symptoms. Simply losing weight around the abdomen improves this condition.

Overeating is another common cause of GERD. The excessive intake of food will result in an over-distention of the stomach. An over-distention of the stomach can result in a reflux of stomach contents into the esophagus. Another simple way of improving GERD in those who overeat is to decrease the portion sizes at meal time.

2. *DRINK WATER*

My clinical experience has clearly shown that dehydration is another common cause of GERD. A traditional Chinese doctor might say that GERD is a result of excess fire in the stomach, rising into the esophagus. What do you put fire out with? Water. I have found that most cases of GERD are associated with inadequate water intake and dehydration. GERD improves when a dehydrated condition is rectified. In a dehydrated state, the stomach will unable to produce the mucous necessary to protect itself and reflux of gastric contents into the esophagus is much more common. Ensuring an adequate water intake (see Table 3 below) will help prevent/treat GERD.

TABLE 3: HOW MUCH WATER TO INGEST
1. Take your weight in pounds. 2. Divide the weight in half. 3. The final number is the number of ounces of water/day.

3. *CHIROPRACTIC CARE FOR GERD*

A simple chiropractic technique of manipulating the gastroesophageal junction has proven effective for many patients.[31] This technique is particularly effective for those with a hiatal hernia as well as overweight individuals. Furthermore, those under undue amounts of stress can benefit from manipulation of the gastroesophageal junction. A skilled chiropractor can assist you with this technique.

4. *ELIMINATE FOOD ALLERGIES WITH ACUPRESSURE*

Food allergies are also a common cause of gastric problems including GERD. My clinical experience has continually shown that the diagnosis and elimination of food allergies has proven to be a crucial part of helping the gastrointestinal system function optimally. Food allergies appear to cause a dysfunction in the LES resulting in a reflux of the gastric contents into the esophagus. If the reflux contents go further up the esophagus, it can irritate the airways resulting in asthma symptoms.

Food allergies have been associated not only with asthma, but with eczema, hay fever and hives. Many of the patients suffering with these conditions also have lowered stomach acid production. An acupressure technique, NAET, has proven extremely helpful at diagnosing and eliminating food and environmental allergies. I have personally treated many patients with GERD (as well as many other conditions) with NAET, and have witnessed many positive results. For more information on NAET, please see the Appendix.

WHAT DO ACID-BLOCKING DRUGS DO?

Acid blocking drugs do what they are designed to do: poison an enzyme (hydrogen/potassium adenosine triphosphatase enzyme system—H^+/K^+ ATPase) of the gastric parietal cell. The end result is that the proton pump cannot secrete acid into the stomach. Without acid production, the pH of the stomach will rise abnormally.

Interfering with the normal acid production of the stomach can have disastrous effects, including sharply increasing the risk of developing cancer, overgrowth of bacteria, yeast, and parasites.

ARE ACID-BLOCKING DRUGS EVER NEEDED?

Yes. Acid-blocking drugs do have their place. In the cases of an active ulcer in the stomach or duodenum, taking a short course ($\approx$1-4 weeks) of acid-blocking drugs can facilitate healing of the mucosa. Also, if the lower esophageal sphincter is damaged or not functioning, acid- blocking drugs may be the only solution.

However, the long-term use of acid-blocking drugs will inevitably lead to more adverse effects. Common sense tells us that poisoning the enzyme in the stomach that produces hydrochloric acid over a long period of time will not be a good thing. The medical literature has clearly shown that the long-term use of acid-blocking drugs is associated with increases of cancer of the stomach as well as serious bacterial infections such as C. difficile.

WHY ARE ACID BLOCKING DRUGS SUCH A PROBLEM?

We eat food in order to provide energy to our bodies. Food needs to be broken down into vitamins, minerals, amino acids, glucose, and other constituents. These items are necessary for optimizing a wide range of physiologic functions as well as producing energy. A good digestive system results in our bodies being able to properly digest food in order to obtain the proper nutrients. This ensures that our bodies will maintain the proper store of vitamins, minerals, and amino acids.

It is impossible to get the proper nutrients out of food if we don't have adequate amounts of hydrochloric acid to begin the digestive process of food. The stomach was designed to produce a large amount of hydrochloric acid for a reason; to digest food. Without adequate amounts of hydrochloric acid, this vital function will be compromised.

As the pH of the stomach rises, the ability of the stomach to properly digest food will decline. Due to the elevated pH, there will be a tendency for overgrowth of abnormal forms of bacteria, parasites, and yeast in the stomach as well as the rest of the gastrointestinal tract. The elevated pH sets off a cascade of gastrointestinal problems. Long-term administration of acid-blocking agents will inevitably lead to the decline of many other crucial body systems due to the multiple nutritional deficiencies that are associated with the use of these substances.

WHAT CONDITIONS MAY BE ASSOCIATED WITH LOWERED STOMACH ACID?

As previously stated, the ads by Big Pharma make us think that stomach acid is bad for you. Big Pharma would have us believe this villain (stomach acid) is responsible for stomach ulcers, gastroesophageal reflux disease, gastritis, and other conditions.

However, adequate amounts of stomach acid play a vital role in many important metabolic processes in the body. Furthermore, a low stomach acid environment will inevitably lead to poor health and the development of chronic disease.

The reason we are designed to eat is to help replenish our store of vital nutrients—vitamins, minerals, amino acids, and enzymes for use in our bodies. If we become deficient in these vital nutrients, it will set the stage for the development of chronic illness.

An adequate amount of stomach acid is necessary for the proper digestion of food. If food is not broken down appropriately, it will lead to nutrient deficiencies. All of the vital nutrients in our bodies, including amino acids, vitamins, minerals, and enzymes are dependant on adequate stomach acid to allow these vital nutrients to be absorbed.

TABLE 4: CONDITIONS ASSOCIATED WITH LOW STOMACH ACID

Acne[32]
Acne Rosacea

Allergies[33]
Asthma[34]
Autoimmune disorders
     Hashimoto's disease
     Graves' disease
     Lupus
     Rheumatoid Arthritis[35 36 37]
Eczema[38]
Hives[39]
Gall Bladder disorders
     Gall stones
     Infection
Leaky gut
Migraines[40]
Vitamin B-12 deficiency

If there is suboptimal production of stomach acid, or if medications that block the production of stomach acid (e.g., Nexium®, Prilosec®, etc.) are used, it will ensure multiple nutritional deficiencies. Table 4 gives examples of the conditions associated with long-term suboptimal production of stomach acid.

ELIMINATING ASTHMA WITH HYDROCHLORIC ACID

Many times asthma is treated with acid-blocking drugs to decrease GERD. Asthma is not an illness caused by a deficiency of acid-blocking drugs. A recent study failed to show any benefit of using a proton pump inhibitor (Nexium) with asthmatic patients.[41]

In fact, research has shown that asthmatic patients generally have a low hydrochloric acid production. Eighty years ago, a physician reported that over eighty percent of 200 asthmatic children had a low stomach acid secretion. Nearly ten percent of those studied had no acid production. The physician placed these children on hydrochloric acid therapy and noticed that most asthmatic symptoms significantly improved.[42]

Furthermore, asthmatic patients can have dramatic improvements in their symptoms by eliminating refined foods from their diets. Refined foods lead to many nutritional deficiencies and will decrease the effectiveness of the lower esophageal sphincter. Eliminating refined foods includes eliminating refined sugar, flour, salt, and oils. For more information on how to eliminate refined foods, I refer the reader to my book, ***The Guide to Healthy Eating.***

John, age 47, suffered with asthma for 40 years. "I was diagnosed as a child and I have been on medicine ever since then," he said. John was being treated with two inhalers to help him control the asthma symptoms. Also, he had trouble exercising due to having shortness of breath. Furthermore, he suffered with many food allergies. "I can tell when I eat food that isn't good for me. My sinuses will get stuffy which triggers the asthma," he claimed. John found that dairy and wheat products seem to be particularly strong triggers. He also complained of a feeling of food sitting in his stomach after he ate. This is a cardinal sign of low stomach acid production. John also had many signs of low hydrochloric acid production on a physical exam including having thinned nails and very dry skin. Due to his symptoms and a Heidelberg test which showed low stomach acid production as well as the physical exam signs, I elected to give John a therapeutic trial of hydrochloric acid supplements. John was instructed to take five grains (300mg) of hydrochloric acid with each meal. If he had a large meal or a meal with meat, he was to take ten grains (600mg) of hydrochloric acid. Within two days, most of his symptoms were gone. "It was unbelievable. I knew things were better after I took the first dose. All of my stomach discomfort is now gone. My asthma symptoms are over 90% better. I don't have to use my medication nearly as much. Even my food allergies are so much better," he claimed.

Many patients with low stomach acid will complain of food sitting in their stomachs for a prolonged period of time. Food allergies are much more common when there is insufficient stomach acid produced. Furthermore, asthmatic patients often improve their condition when appropriately supplemented with hydrochloric acid. Many gastrointestinal complaints can be rectified with the use of hydrochloric acid supplementation.

PUTTING IT ALL TOGETHER: ADEQUATE STOMACH ACID IS VITAL TO HEALTH

Stomach acid was given to us for a reason; to help with the digestion of food. If we interfere with the production of stomach acid, it will lead to poor health. Before instituting therapy with a drug that poisons an enzyme which makes stomach acid, why not have your stomach acid levels measured first? You will be surprised at the findings; more often low stomach acid levels will be present, not high stomach acid levels. This can be performed with a simple, out-patient test known as a Heidelberg test. I have been doing this test in my office for years.

Good digestion starts in the stomach. This begins with the adequate production of stomach acid. We should be supporting the natural physiology of the body, not poisoning it.

FINAL THOUGHTS

Low stomach acid production is a major health problem. The long-term use of acid-blocking drugs will result in a poor digestive system and many vitamin and mineral deficiencies. This will eventually lead to serious issues such as atrophic gastritis and cancers of the gastrointestinal tract. We should work to maintain adequate stomach acid production; not inhibit it. It only makes sense. Stomach acid is produced for a reason; to help you properly digest your food. *Remember, you can't poison a crucial enzyme or block an important receptor for the long-term and expect a good result.*

[1] Yamada, T. Clinical relevance of GI hormones: Emerging interest in hypergastrinemia. Ann. of Int. Med.2.15.93. Vol. 118, Issue 4. p.309-311

[2] Winsett, O. Gastrin stimulates growth of colon cancer. Surgery. 1986;99:302-307

[3] Tadatka, Y. IBID.

[4] Peterson, W. Role of H. pylori in gastric acid secretion and serum gastrin concentrations in healthy subjects and patients with duodenal ulcer. Gastroent. 1991;100:A140

[5] Bernard, MA. The effect of vitamin B12 deficiency on older veterans and its relationship to health. J. Am. Geriat. Soc. 1998:46:1199-206

[6] Sato, Y. Effect of folate and methylcobalamin on hip fractures in patients with stroke. JAMA. 2005. 293;182-8

[7] Herbert, V. Vitamin B12 in present knowledge in nutrition. 17th ed. International Life Institute Press. 1996

[8] Healton, EB. Neurological aspects of cobalamin deficiency. Medicine 1991;70:229-244

[9] Bottiglieri T. Folate, vitamin B12, and neuropsychiatric disorders. Nutr Rev 1996;54:382-90.

[10] American Medical News. June 8, 2009

[11] The Economist. May 27, 2006.

[12] FP News. 9.15.06

[13] FP News. 9.15.06. Numbers extrapolated from the 6 states reported.

[14] The Economist. May 27, 2006 and CDC.

[15] Dial, S. Use of gastric acid suppressive agents and the risk of community acquired clostridium difficile associated diseases. JAMA. 2005;294:2989-2995

[16] Bock OAA, et al: The serum pepsinogen level with special reference to the histology of the gastric mucosa. Gut 1953, 4: 106-111

[17] Varis K, et al: An appraisal of tests for severe atrophic gastritis in relatives of patients with pernicious anemia. Dig.Dis. Sci. 1979, 24: 187-191

[18] Kazumasa, M. Serum pepsinogen as a screening test of extensive chronic gastritis. Gastroenterologia Japanica. Vol. 22., No. 2. 1987

[19] Demiroglu H, Dundar S: Pernicious anaemia patients should be screened for iron deficiency during follow up. N Z Med J 1997 Apr 25; 110(1042): 147-8

[20] N.Eng. J. Med. 2006;354:1787-95

[21] CDC. Accessed 5.5.06: www.cdc.gov/ulcer/md.htm

[22] CDC. IBID. Accessed 5.05.06.

[23] Al-Habbal, MF. A double blind controlled clinical trial of mastic and placebo in the treatment of duodenal ulcer. Clin. Exp. Pharm. Physiol. 1984. Sep-Oct;11(5):541-4

[24] CDC. IBID. Accessed 5.5.06

[25] Huwez, Fu. Mastic gum kills H. pylori. N. Eng. J. Med. 1998, 339;1946

[26] Odashima, M. Induciton of a 72-kDa heat-shock protein in cultured rat gastric mucosal cells and rat gastric mucosa by zinc L-carnosine. Dig. Dis. Sci. 2002. Dec;47(12):2799-2804

[27] Matsukura, T. Applicability of zinc complex of L-carnosine for medical use. Biochemisty (Moxc). 2000.Jul;65(7):817-23

[28] Ishihara, R. Polaprezinc attenuates H. pylori associated gastritis in Mongolian gerbils. Helicobacter. 2002. Dec;7(6):384-9

[29] Lin, Yt. Inhibition of H. pylori and associated urease by oregano and cranberry photochemical synergies. Appl. Environ. Microbiol. 2005. Dec;71(12):8558-64

[30] Digestive Diseases in the United States: Epidemiology and Impact, National Digestive Diseases Data Working Group, James E. Everhart, MD, MPH, Editor, US Department of Health and Human Services, Public Health Service, National Institutes of Health, NIH Publication No. 94-1447, May 1994

[31] Barral, J. Visceral Manipulation. 1983

[32] Knowles, F. Gastric acidity and acne vulgaris. Arch. Erm. Syphilogy. 1926, 13:215

[33] Bray, G. The hypochlorhydria of asthma in childhood. Quart. J. Med. 1931, 24:181

[34] Bray, G. The hypochlorhydria of asthma in childhood. Quart. J. Med. 1931, 24:181

[35] Woodward, A. The relation of the gastric secretion to rheumatoid arthritis. Lancet, Oct 5, 1912;942-5

[36] de Witte, TJ. Hypochlorhydria and hypergastrinaemia in rheumatoid arthritis. Ann. Rheum. Dis. 1979, 38:14-7

[37] Marcolongo, R. Gastrointestinal involvement in rheumatoid arthritis.: A biopsy study. J. Rheum. 1979, 6:163-73

[38] Bray, G. IBID. 1931

[39] Bray, G. IBID. 1931

[40] Bray, G. IBID. 1931

[41] N. Eng. J. of Med. 2009;360:1487-99

[42] Bray, G. IBID. 1931

Chapter 7

Antidepressant Drugs

INTRODUCTION

Who hasn't seen an ad for an antidepressant medication? Since the 1980's when Prozac® was released and marketed by Eli Lilly, we have been inundated with ads touting the benefits of the antidepressant medications. Big Pharma has been trying to convince all of us that we need antidepressant medications to help us improve our lifestyles. Presently, one in ten American women take an antidepressant drug. The use of antidepressant drugs has tripled over the past decade.[1] The National Institute of Mental Health (NIMH) claims that 26.2% of the adult U.S. population currently suffers from a diagnosable mental disorder.[2] Mood disorders (e.g., depression) are the most common form of mental disorders present. The NIMH estimates that 95% of the adult U.S. population currently suffers from a mood disorder.[3]

Over the last 30 years, the number of diagnoses for mood disorders has increased exponentially. Why would there be such an increase in mental disorders? If you were trying to increase the number of people taking a drug, the first step is to give them a diagnosis that will require a drug to treat it. There is no question that people are being over-diagnosed with mental disorders and over-treated with antidepressant medications.

Susan, age 52, had not felt well for years. She said, "I don't know what happened. I haven't felt good for a long time." Susan had seen various doctors and was told nothing was wrong with her. The last two doctors had recommended that she see a psychiatrist and take an antidepressant medication. She was prescribed an antidepressant medication (Prozac®) by a psychiatrist who spent ten minutes with her. "He did not even touch me or listen to my heart. I felt he had his mind made up before I walked in the door," Susan claimed. She tried the antidepressant medication but did not like the side effects. "The medication made me a zombie. I could not think straight and it caused me to be nervous," she said. When I saw Susan, I took a detailed history, performed a physical exam, and ordered laboratory tests. I diagnosed Susan with fibromyalgia—a condition that is characterized by fatigue and body aches. When I took a dietary history from Susan, it was clear that she was eating a poor diet, full of refined, devitalized food. Testing also found Susan to be very low in many amino acids as well as many vitamins and minerals. Finally, Susan was dehydrated. She was drinking 2-4 diet sodas per day and two cups of coffee (with Equal®) per day. I educated Susan about good food choices and had her meet with my nutritionist. I recommended amino acid supplements (5-HTP and tyrosine) as well as a comprehensive nutritional program including vitamins and minerals. I also advised her to avoid artificial sweeteners and use water as her beverage-of-choice. One month later, Susan reported, "I can't believe how much better I feel. My family is even commenting on how I am so much happier."

There is an old saying I frequently remind my patients of: Garbage in equals garbage out. Eating a healthier diet is the most important factor in improving anyone's health. The number one reason people aren't feeling well is because they are eating a poor diet. Eating a poor diet will ensure that the body will not function optimally. Just as you would not put poor quality gas in your automobile, it is not smart to put poor quality food in your body. Poor quality food will lead to multiple nutritional imbalances, as evidenced in Susan's case. How are our brains supposed to make the proper neurotransmitters if the basic raw materials are not being supplied to the body? Susan did not have an 'antidepressant medication deficiency condition'; she had multiple nutritional imbalances that caused her ill feelings. I have seen countless patients improve a depressed condition by doing the basics; cleaning up the diet, avoiding artificial sweeteners, and drinking adequate amounts of water. More information on a healthy diet can be found in ***The Guide To Healthy Eating.***

INTRODUCTION TO SELECTIVE SEROTONIN REUPTAKE INHIBITORS: SSRI's

Although there are a plethora of mental health drugs currently on the market, this chapter will focus on the most common antidepressants, the selective serotonin reuptake inhibitiors (SSRI's). SSRI's have become the most commonly prescribed antidepressant drugs in the U.S. over the last ten years. Examples of SSRI's include: Prozac®, Zoloft®, Paxil®, Lexapro®, and Celexa®. In 2004, there were 26 million prescriptions for Lexapro dispensed.[4] With the increasing numbers of mental health disorder diagnoses, children as well as adults are being prescribed this class of drugs for an ever widening array of complaints.

What is serotonin? What are the SSRI's? How do they work? Are they effective? Are there alternatives? These questions will be answered throughout this chapter.

WHAT IS HOMEOSTASIS?

From the beginning of medical school I was taught about homeostasis. Homeostasis refers to the living organism trying to regulate its internal environment in order to maintain a steady physiologic state. For example, if it is cold outside, the body will increase the heat production to keep itself warm. Conversely, in a hot environment, the body may sweat in order to cool itself off.

The brain also works to try and maintain homeostasis. During a stressful situation, the brain will increase the production of certain neurotransmitters (adrenaline) and hormones (noradrenaline) to help the body respond to the stress. During relaxation, other neurotransmitters (serotonin) and hormones (melatonin) are produced to help the body relax.

Remember, the brain and the body are always working to achieve homeostasis. As mentioned above, when there is undue stress, the brain responds to the stress by releasing stress neurotransmitters and stress hormones. This is an appropriate response. If we need to run or if we need to fight, it is appropriate for an increased production of norepinephrine and epinephrine. We would be inhibited from running or fighting if we did not have enough of these powerful chemicals being produced and utilized. After the stressful event has subsided, the brain still desires to be in homeostasis. As the production of the stress chemicals decline normal function will resume and the body will again restore homeostasis.

WHAT CAN DISRUPT HOMEOSTASIS?

Many things can disrupt the brain's ability to maintain homeostasis. Nutritional deficiencies can disrupt many vital functions in the body, including the maintenance of homeostasis. When there are vitamin and mineral deficiencies, the body will be unable to create the precursors necessary for the adequate production of neurotransmitters and hormones. If the body does not have the basic raw materials to manufacture the substances it desires, homeostasis cannot be maintained. The end result of these deficiencies is the onset of chronic illness such as depression, anxiety, ADHD, cancer, and fatigue.

Drugs can also disrupt the brain's ability to achieve and maintain homeostasis. Drugs that block receptors or poison enzymes will, by their nature, disrupt the normal functioning of the body. The end result of many drug therapies is an inability of the body to achieve and maintain homeostasis.

The most commonly used antidepressant drugs all block receptors or poison enzymes in the brain, as well as in other tissues in the body. For the SSRI's, the substance that is most commonly disrupted is serotonin. As mentioned previously, ***it is*** ***impossible to achieve your optimal health by poisoning a crucial*** ***enzyme or blocking an important receptor for the long-term.***

WHAT IS SEROTONIN?

Our brains are made up of chemicals called neurotransmitters. Neurotransmitters are the substances produced in the brain that allow it to do all of the functions that the brain was designed to do including thinking, feeling, mood regulation, sleep control, hunger, satiety, and more. The brain cannot function without an adequate supply and balance of neurotransmitters. In fact, life is not compatible without an adequate supply of neurotransmitters. Serotonin is a neurotransmitter. Table 1 shows you some examples of neurotransmitters found in the brain.

```
┌─────────────────────────────────────────────────┐
│ TABLE 1:  EXAMPLES OF NEUROTRANSMITTERS          │
│                                                  │
│ Adrenaline                                       │
│ Dopamine                                         │
│ Histamine                                        │
│ Noradrenaline                                    │
│ Serotonin                                        │
└─────────────────────────────────────────────────┘
```

Serotonin is produced from the amino acid tryptophan (see Figure 1). Recall that amino acids are the basic building blocks of the body. In fact, all of the neurotransmitters (e.g., noradrenaline, adrenaline, dopamine) are made from their basic building blocks: amino acids. Further discussion of amino acids and their relationship to neurotransmitter deficiency will be discussed later in this chapter.

```
┌─────────────────────────────────────────────────┐
│                                                  │
│          Figure 1:  Production of Serotonin      │
│                                                  │
│                                                  │
│  Tryptophan──►5-hydroxy-tryptophan ──► Serotonin │
│                    (5-HTP)                        │
│                                                  │
│                                                  │
└─────────────────────────────────────────────────┘
```

Serotonin is responsible for learning and the regulation of sleep and mood. It is known as one of the 'feel good' neurotransmitters. Serotonin is found throughout the entire brain. More serotonin is produced and utilized in the brain than any of the other neurotransmitters. In fact, serotonin can regulate and control the effects of the other neurotransmitters.[5]

205

The adult human body contains approximately 5-10mg of serotonin, however, only ten percent of the body's serotonin is found in the brain.

What is less well known is that nearly 90% of the body's serotonin stores are in the intestinal tract, where it plays a critical role in the digestion process.[6] In addition, serotonin also helps regulate the contraction and expansion of the blood vessels of the body and also regulates the function of the platelets. Although all of the neurotransmitters help regulate different behaviors, through a complex set of interactions that is unknown today, certain traits appear to be primarily controlled by serotonin. Table 2 gives some of the behaviors and functions serotonin is thought to regulate.[7]

Table 2: Behaviors Regulated by Serotonin

Appetite
Alcohol and nicotine cravings
Drug abuse
Gastrointestinal effects
Heart and blood flow
Impulse control and aggression
Mental Functioning
Migraine and other headaches
Mood
Motivation
Sleep-wake cycle

Serotonin, like all of the other neurotransmitters, is released by a cell at a synapse. A synapse is a tiny space between two cells where the pre-synaptic cell releases a substance that binds with its receptor on the post-synaptic cell. This binding with the post-synaptic cell results in the post-synaptic cell becoming active and performing whatever its function is supposed to be. In the brain, the activity may be a thought or an emotion. It is known that serotonin can affect many different areas of the brain by binding to its receptors. However, the effect of serotonin is not consistent between different individuals. In some, it may cause happiness; in others sadness.

According to Big Pharma, serotonin deficiency is thought to underlie many cases of depression. Big Pharma has created a whole class of medications that poison an important enzyme in order to promote higher serotonin levels in the brain. As previously mentioned, the most common antidepressant drugs in use today--SSRI's--such as Prozac®, Zoloft®, and Paxil®, are part of a class of antidepressants called selective serotonin reuptake inhibitors.

In order for the cells of the brain to communicate with one another, there has to be adequate amounts of all of the neurotransmitters. The brain cannot think, feel, keep us alert, or perform any of its vital functions without the optimal production and ratio of neurotransmitters.

WHAT ARE THE SSRI'S?

The $\underline{S}$elective $\underline{S}$erotonin $\underline{R}$euptake $\underline{I}$nhibitors (SSRI's) are a class of antidepressant medications. SSRI's are the most widely prescribed psychiatric medications and generate billions of dollars in sales. They have largely replaced the older class of antidepressant medications such as the tricyclic antidepressants. According to Big Pharma, the SSRI's were developed to lessen the side effects associated with the older classes of antidepressants. Furthermore, the newer classes of antidepressants were touted as more effective than the older classes of medications. Of course, the older medications were off-patent and the newer SSRI's have current patents which makes them more expensive. Unfortunately, the research has shown that the SSRI's are neither more effective nor have fewer side effects as compared to the older class of antidepressants.

The ads for the antidepressants claim that antidepressant medications, especially SSRI's, effectively treat imbalances in the neurotransmitters. In the case of the SSRI's (e.g., Prozac®, Paxil®, and Zoloft®), the imbalance is assumed to be serotonin. The imbalance is generally referred to as a serotonin deficiency. It is interesting that patients are being told they have a serotonin imbalance or a chemical imbalance in their brain even though they have never had their serotonin levels measured.

Brain function is not well understood. We know that there is electrical activity of the brain and this electrical activity is governed in part from the neurotransmitters. This electrical activity causes serotonin to be released from the nerve cell. This nerve cell is called the presynaptic cell. After its release, serotonin binds to its receptor, completing the transmission of the impulse. When serotonin binds to that receptor, it electrically stimulates the postsynaptic cell.

Once serotonin binds to the postsynaptic cell its job is completed. Our body has designed a system in order to ensure the brain does not get too much stimulation from serotonin. Once serotonin has stimulated the postsynaptic cell, it is reabsorbed back into the presynaptic cell for future use.

This reabsorption process is very important. It is one of the many control points that the brain has to ensure proper function and homeostasis.

Let's look at what would happen if serotonin were not reabsorbed. If serotonin were not reabsorbed, it would constantly stimulate the postsynaptic receptor. This constant stimulation can cause many problems such as nervousness, anxiety, hyper-responsiveness. Serotonin syndrome is a serious condition whereby excess serotonin is over stimulating the brain.[8] Serotonin syndrome is an adverse effect of many common antidepressants, particularly the SSRI's (e.g., Prozac®, Paxil®, and Zoloft®). All of the SSRI's poison the enzyme that is responsible for reabsorbing serotonin at its receptor. Cocaine is a substance that works under a similar mechanism as the SSRI's by blocking the reuptake of certain neurotransmitters (e.g., dopamine) resulting in a heightened state.

Big Pharma would have you believe that low levels of neurotransmitters such as serotonin and/or dopamine are the underlying cause(s) of depression. Therefore, Big Pharma's logic would dictate that in order to elevate the low levels, you need a drug that blocks the reuptake of the neurotransmitter(s).

However, Big Pharma's logic does not make sense. We must keep in mind that depression is not an illness that is caused by an 'antidepressant medication deficiency'. If someone is deficient in a neurotransmitter, then why not supplement with the agent necessary to increase the neurotransmitter?   Or, perhaps change the diet in order to supply the body with the raw materials to produce the neurotransmitter. Further information on diet can be found in ***The Guide to Healthy Eating.***

Serotonin reuptake inhibitors have been studied for over 25 years.   Although Big Pharma would have you believe otherwise, little is known about much of the effects of serotonin (or the other neurotransmitters) in the brain. Big Pharma gives doctors seminars and glossy brochures telling them the virtues of blocking the reuptake of serotonin in the brain.   As stated previously, over 90% of the body's serotonin is produced <u>outside</u> of the brain. What are the consequences of blocking the reuptake of serotonin outside of the brain? No one knows. There has not been a lot of interest in this question.

There are a multitude of adverse effects of SSRI's—see Table 3 (page 213). ***Remember, you can't poison a crucial enzyme for the long-term and expect a good result.*** I believe the large number of adverse effects of the SSRI's is secondary to the poisoning of a crucial enzyme that is responsible for maintaining the correct balance of serotonin in the brain. In the individual, it is impossible to predict what the outcome will be when this enzyme is poisoned.

ARE THE ANTIDEPRESSANTS MORE EFFECTIVE THAN A PLACEBO? ARE NEWER ANTIDEPRESSANTS MORE EFFECTIVE THAN OLDER ANTIDEPRESSANTS?

When all of the studies of the seven newest antidepressants (Prozac®, Zoloft®, Paxil®, Effexor®, Serzone®, Remeron®, and Welbutron SR®) were reviewed in 2000, researchers found surprising results. These blockbuster antidepressant medications were not found to be significantly more effective than a placebo.[9] In fact, the placebo was found to improve the symptoms of depression by 30.9% while those that took the antidepressants listed above improved the symptoms of depression by 40.7%. Furthermore, the older antidepressants, the tricyclics (e.g., Elavil®, and Pamelor®) were found to be 41.7%

effective in treating the symptoms of depression—just as effective as the newer SSRI's.

So, why are the SSRI's so widely prescribed? Clever advertising and marketing has made the SSRI's a huge success for Big Pharma. A 40% success rate--that is barely above the placebo rate--should not be celebrated. Certainly, with their high rate of adverse effects including suicide, other methods to treat depression should be investigated and utilized.

THE ADVERSE EFFECTS ASSOCIATED WITH ANTIDEPRESSANT MEDICATIONS

Antidepressants are responsible for a wide range of adverse effects. Table 3, compiled by Dr. Peter Bregin, author of **_The Antidepressant Fact Book_** (Perseus Publishing) provides a list of the frequency of some of the most common adverse effects of Prozac.[10] Dr. Bregin claims the pharmaceutical company that makes the block-buster drug Prozac®, Eli Lilly, obscures the dangers of Prozac® by putting the adverse effects in many different places in the package insert. He meticulously went through the insert and compiled all the adverse effects into one chart—Table 3. When one looks at the rate of adverse effects of Prozac®, the frequency of problems associated with Prozac® is astounding. In fact, many of the adverse effects Prozac® are strikingly similar to the depressed conditions Prozac is supposed to treat.

TABLE 3: FREQUENCY OF ADVERSE EFFECTS OF PROZAC

Agitation	frequent
Amnesia	frequent
Anxiety	12-15%
Dizziness	10%
Insomnia	16-33%
Libido Decreased	3-11%
Somnolence	13-17%
Tremors	10%

If Table 3 were not enough to caution you about using an SSRI, a new study showed that the overall risk of dying is 55% higher if you take an antidepressant.[11] [12] In this study, subjects were followed for three years. At the end of the study, 21.4% of the patients taking antidepressants had died compared to 12.5% of those not taking antidepressants. The death rate at the end of the study is known as the all-cause mortality. It is rare for studies funded by Big Pharma to report all-cause mortality rates at the end of their drug-funded studies. If they did, many drugs would lose much of their luster. *Remember, you can't poison a crucial enzyme for the long-term and expect a good outcome.*

Maternal use of SSRI's has been linked to an increased risk of neonatal hypertension. Infants of women who took SSRI's in the second half of pregnancy were five to six times more likely to develop persistent pulmonary hypertension of the newborn (PPHN). The reported incidence of PPHN was 1 case for every 100 exposed infants.[13] Infants exposed to SSRI's, had a ten-fold higher risk of PPHN as compared to infants not exposed to SSRI's.

ANTIDEPRESSANTS AND SUICIDE

Big Pharma advertises antidepressant medications as an effective tool to help people overcome depression. These drugs are even being promoted as effective agents for children. Suicidal thoughts and behavior frequently accompany severe depression. The FDA has issued a Public Health Advisory about the relationship of antidepressants and suicide. This Public Health Advisory states:[14]

1. Adults being treated with antidepressant medicines, particularly those being treated for depression, should be watched closely for worsening of depression and for increased suicidal thinking or behavior.

2. Close observation of adults may be especially important when antidepressant medications are started for the first time or when doses for the specific drugs prescribed have been changed.

3. Adults whose symptoms worsen while being treated with antidepressants, including an increase in suicidal thinking or behavior, should be evaluated by their health care professional.

I was taught in medical school that suicidal behavior could be treated with antidepressant medications. The FDA advisory would lead one to think that antidepressant drugs may in fact be causing suicidal behavior in a depressed individual.

CHILDREN, ANTIDEPRESSANTS AND SUICIDE

Adults may not be the only people at risk for increases in suicide while on antidepressants. Children treated with antidepressants may also have an increased risk of suicide. A recent study found there was a 52 % increase in suicide attempts in children and adolescents who were treated with an antidepressant medication as compared to a similar group of depressed children and adolescents not treated with an antidepressant drug. Furthermore, this same study found that children and adolescents treated with an antidepressant drug were 15 times more likely to die of the attempt as compared to children with depression but not treated with an antidepressant.[15] This study did not show a similar correlation with adults treated with antidepressant medications.

A trial comparing Paxil with the older antidepressant medication Clomipramine (a member of the older tricyclic antidpressant medications) in adolescents found that 75% of those studied had an adverse reaction on Paxil.[16] This included one in eight--13%--committing a suicidal act.

215

Do antidepressants increase or decrease the suicide rate? There are studies that support both sides of this argument. However, until this argument is cleared up, I feel that antidepressant medications should be used only in an emergent condition or as a last resort, after other nontoxic therapies have been exhausted.

The number of children treated with psychotropic drugs, including antidepressants and stimulants, has increased at an exponential rate over the last ten years. The number of two to four year olds on psychotropic drugs jumped over 50% between 1991 and 1995.[17] These numbers have continued to dramatically increase since then. In fact, there are estimated to be over seven million antidepressant prescriptions filled for children less than 18 years of age.[18]

How much have the drugs been researched in children? Very little. We don't know the developmental consequences of putting children on these powerful and dangerous drugs. I believe drug therapies should be a last resort for children and adolescents. Unfortunately, that is not the case today. Children are given prescriptions for stimulants and antidepressants at routine, short office visits. There is very little monitoring of adverse effects. There are safer therapies, such as psychotherapy and excercise, that should be investigated first.

IS PSYCHOTHERAPY AN EFFECTIVE TOOL FOR DEPRESSION?

What other tools besides drugs can be used to help someone overcome depression? Psychotherapy, with an experienced practitioner can be a very effective tool to treat depression. Psychotherapy is a set of techniques that help improve mental health including emotional and behavioral issues. Psychotherapy helps to clarify the relationship between the conscious and the unconscious realms.[19]

A large study funded by the National Institute of Mental Health compared psychotherapy to antidepressant drugs.[20] At the end of sixteen weeks of treatment, there was little difference in efficacy between psychotherapy and drug treatment for depression. Similar results have been seen in other studies.[21] [22] [23] [24] [25]

However, psychotherapy is not plagued with the adverse effects that antidepressant medications are prone to. Psychotherapy can take longer than antidepressant mediations to work—6-8 weeks for psychotherapy as compared to 1-6 weeks for drugs. [26] [27] Psychotherapy can be an effective tool to help the patient understand the underlying cause of depression and develop mechanisms to reverse the underlying cause and prevent depression in the future.

Although I do not have personal experience with psychotherapy, there is no question that I have seen improvements in my patients at the hands of a clinician experienced with utilizing psychotherapy.

EXERCISE AND DEPRESSION

An interesting study looked at comparing exercise as a treatment modality versus antidepressant drugs in treating major depression.[28] Researchers designed the study with three groups: a group treated with exercise, a group treated with exercise and Zoloft® and a group treated with Zoloft® alone. After four months of treatment, depression significantly improved in all three groups. However, relapse of depression occurred in 38% of those treated with Zoloft® and 31% of those treated with Zoloft® and exercise. Those in the exercise only group had an 8% recurrence of depression. This study accomplished a relapse rate of only 8% without the use of an expensive drug that has numerous side effects. No psychotropic drug therapy has demonstrated this positive effect without any risk of adverse effects.

Exercise has been shown to raise serotonin levels. This exercise-induced elevation of serotonin levels can help many who suffer from depression. Exercise is certainly less expensive and has a lot less toxicity as compared to an antidepressant medication. I can only wonder why this study did not make headlines across the country. I have seen wonderful effects in my patients who begin an exercise program. An exercise program can include simply walking. If you are not in good shape, start with walking five minutes per day. Gradually increase the walking until you can do at least 30 minutes. My clinical experience has shown that walking or some form of exercise that lasts at least 30 minutes per day can improve depression and mood in nearly everyone.

THE CASE FOR EATING A CLEAN DIET

Unfortunately, physicians that are prescribing the antidepressant medications for their patients are rarely concerned about the diet of their patients. In medical school, obtaining and evaluating a dietary history as well as giving dietary advice was not emphasized.

My experience has been clear: improving one's diet can certainly improve nearly all illnesses including depression. Food is supposed to supply the body with the basic raw materials including vitamins, minerals, and enzymes. These basic raw materials are used to manufacture amino acids, proteins and neurotransmitters that allow the brain as well as the rest of the body to optimally function.

For the long-term, eating a diet deficient in these raw materials will lead to a deficiency of the basic items that our brain (and body) requires to function optimally.

I believe that an imbalance of the brain's neurotransmitters often stems from a poor diet. A poor diet will lead to multiple nutritional deficiencies. How is the brain supposed to manufacture an adequate serotonin (or any other neurotransmitter) level if it doesn't have the raw materials available to it?

Which foods lead to a poor diet? The 'whites' are the biggest culprits. The 'whites' refer to white sugar, white flour, and white salt. Each of these items is a devitalized food that has had all of its minerals and enzymes removed in order to prolong the shelf life. Everybody can improve their health by avoiding the 'whites'. However, there is more urgency for someone who is suffering from a chronic illness such as depression to clean up their diet. Eating food devoid of nutrients will cause our body to use its own nutrient store to aid in the digestion process. The long-term ingestion of devitalized food will result in multiple nutritional deficiencies and the onset and worsening of chronic illness.

Furthermore, the ingestion of excess amounts of the 'whites' will lead to blood sugar abnormalities. Long-term ingestion of the 'whites' will cause an elevation of blood sugar, eventually causing diabetes. We are in the midst of an epidemic of adult onset diabetes that is being driven from the excess ingestion of the 'whites'. The 'whites' not only cause blood sugar abnormalities; they also lead to depletion of the brain neurotransmitters, particularly serotonin.

I know it can seem daunting to avoid the 'whites'. You don't have to ingest the 'whites'. Refined sugar can be substituted with organic cane sugar or xylitol. Refined grains can be replaced with organic whole grain flour. Refined salt can be substituted with unrefined salt (e.g., Celtic Sea Salt®). Each of these food items contains the basic raw materials that our bodies need. Remember, you are what you eat. For more information on how to make better food choices, I refer the reader to ***The Guide for Healthy Eating*** and ***Salt Your Way To Health.***

RAISING SEROTONIN LEVELS THROUGH DIET AND AMINO ACID SUPPLEMENTATION: THE NATURAL ANTIDEPRSSANT TREATMENT

The food that you eat can influence the levels of all of the neurotransmitters in the body including serotonin. The Standard American Diet (SAD diet) which consists of too many refined foods that lack basic nutrients is a devitalized diet. It leaves many people sad because it depletes the body of the ability to manufacture serotonin and other important neurotransmitters.

Serotonin is not found in appreciable amounts in most food. However the precursor to serotonin, tryptophan, can be found in many different foods. Recall from Figure 1 that tryptophan can be converted into serotonin in the body. A deficiency of tryptophan will lead to a deficiency of serotonin. The SAD diet is full of foods that are low in tryptophan. Corn, the most commonly used grain, contains little tryptophan. Furthermore, most refined breads, pasta and cereals, the staple of the SAD diet, are generally made from grains deficient in

221

tryptophan. Table 4 shows examples of foods that can result in depleted serotonin levels. On the other hand, eating a healthy diet can provide the body with all of the essential ingredients (e.g., tryptophan) to make adequate serotonin as well as other neurotransmitters.

TABLE 4: FOOD THAT CAN RESULT IN DEPLETED SEROTONIN LEVELS
Aspartame Bread (from refined products) Corn Caffeinated Soda Cereal Pasta (from refined products)

As previously stated, nearly all of the neurotransmitters are produced from the body's basic building blocks; amino acids. In the case of serotonin, adequate amounts of the amino acid tryptophan are necessary to produce serotonin. Big Pharma would have you believe that if you are low in serotonin, you should take a drug that poisons an enzyme that helps to reuptake serotonin. *Remember, you can't poison a crucial enzyme or block an important receptor in the body for the long term and expect a good result.*

As shown in this chapter and in the medical research, SSRI's have a tremendous amount of adverse effects. There are better ways to naturally help the body increase its own production of serotonin without having to use toxic medications that are prone to adverse effects.

Since the precursor to serotonin is an amino acid, tryptophan, wouldn't it make sense to check for a deficiency in an amino acid (e.g., tryptophan) before starting a drug that poisons an enzyme? Measuring the levels of the amino acids in the body (via urine testing) is a cost effective way to determine if adequate amounts of the precursors to the neurotransmitters are available.

If amino acids are deficient, how can we raise amino acid levels? Amino acids are supplied in our diet by protein. One of the most common nutritional deficiencies that I see in my practice is an insufficient intake of good protein in the diet. Protein is the best source of amino acids for our bodies. Protein from animal sources contain the largest amount of amino acids of any food group.

The source of protein will have an effect on the quality of the amino acids present. If the animals are fed low-tryptophan containing foods such as corn, the resulting food products will contain suboptimal levels of tryptophan. On the other hand, animals fed and raised in an organic environment will produce more tryptophan in their food products. When animals are fed a healthier diet, the end product (e.g., meat, egg, milk, etc.,) will contain much healthier nutrients in its food.

Organic sources of protein will contain a larger and more diverse content of amino acids as compared to conventionally raised animals. Eggs are the best sources of protein as they are the only food that contains a full complement of all of the essential amino acids necessary for our bodies. Organic eggs have a better supply of nutrients for our bodies than conventional eggs. The same holds true for nearly all food products; organic foods have a more favorable nutrient profile as compared to conventional food products. Table 5 gives some examples of foods that are high in tryptophan.

TABLE 5: FOODS THAT ARE HIGH IN TRYPTOPHAN

Beef
Chicken
Dairy products
Eggs
Nuts
Pork
Pumpkin Seeds
Turkey
Venison

Vegetarian diets are commonly deficient in protein. Vegetarians must take particular care to ensure an adequate intake of protein that contains all of the essential amino acids needed by the body. I encourage vegetarians to do a careful study and think about how to diversify their diet in order to ensure an adequate and balanced protein intake. Working with a health professional knowledgeable about this topic can be extremely helpful for someone eating or considering a change to a vegetarian diet.

IMPROVING DIGESTION TO HELP WITH SEROTONIN PRODUCTION

Some people take in adequate amounts of good sources of protein, yet still have low amino acid levels on testing. How could that be?

Amino acids are the building blocks of the body. They are the precursors to the neurotransmitters. A common cause of amino acid deficiency is a poor digestive process that leads to inadequate protein digestion and therefore, suboptimal amino acid assimilation.

One of the most common causes of inadequate protein digestion is low stomach acid production. The stomach produces a large amount of hydrochloric acid to help properly digest food. How common is low stomach acid production? Unfortunately, very common.

What are people frequently going to their doctors for? Stomach upset, burning in their stomach, reflux esophagitis and more. What does a patient generally get from their doctor? A drug that poisons an enzyme that is responsible for the production of stomach acid. See chapter 6 for more information on antacid drugs.

Antacid drugs are effective at significantly lowering or eliminating stomach acid production. One of the consequences of taking these drugs for the long-term will be poor protein digestion. We have stomach acid for a reason; to help us properly digest protein and absorb amino acids from our food. Long-term uses of antacid drugs need to be avoided.

As people age, they produce less stomach acid. I have seen many patients with suboptimal amino acid levels significantly improve their condition when properly supplemented with hydrochloric acid pills (for more information please see chapter 6).

HOW TO USE FOOD TO ELEVATE SEROTONIN LEVELS

Food can be used to elevate serotonin in the body. Food generally does not contain significant amounts of serotonin or its immediate precursor 5-HTP. The body can convert the amino acid tryptophan into serotonin (see Figure 1, page 205). In fact, tryptophan can cross the blood brain barrier to enter the brain and facilitate the serotonin production process. Tryptophan is supplied from high protein food. Table 5 (page 224) gives some examples of food high in tryptophan. Conventionally raised animals have significantly less serotonin in their meat than organically (or wild) raised animals. Conventionally raised animals are primarily fed with low tryptophan containing grains such as corn or soy. On the other hand, organic farmers will primarily raise their animals with grasses and other plants that the animals were meant to be raised on. These natural foods provide the correct nutrients for the animals which makes their meat much healthier to ingest.

Chronic alcohol use can act as a depressant to the brain and deplete neurotransmitters. The long-term use of large amounts of alcohol will often lead to many nutritional deficiencies and depression. Mild alcohol usage does not seem to cause nutritional deficiencies.

DRINK WATER

I have seen countless patients over the years who complained of depressed symptoms. I always take a dietary history when I am seeing my patients. Part of that dietary history involves finding out which substances are ingested. In asking people what they drink during the day, I am always amazed at how many of the depressed patients are dehydrated.

We all have running water in our homes. How could someone be dehydrated in today's world? It is simple; people are not drinking enough water. People drink too many caffeinated and artificially flavored drinks. These drinks not only supply items that are not healthy for our body (e.g., artificial sweeteners or refined sugar), they actually can make a dehydrated situation worse. Our body is made up of 70% water and the brain is made up of 80% water. I have seen many patients improve a depressed condition by simply rehydrating their body with water. Table 6 gives you recommendations on how much water to ingest.

TABLE 6: HOW MUCH WATER TO INGEST
1. Weight in pounds: _____
2. Divide the weight in pounds by two
3. The answer is the amount of water to ingest in ounces

I cannot stress enough the importance of maintaining good hydration. Maintaining adequate hydration supplies the basic building blocks for a healthy immune system and for maintaining good brain function. I see the positive results of maintaining adequate hydration in my patients every day.

AVOID ASPARTAME

The most commonly used artificial sweetener, Aspartame can disrupt the body's production of serotonin. Aspartame (i.e., Nutrasweet®) contains two excitatory amino acids, phenylalanine and aspartic acid. Both of these amino acids can convert to the stimulatory neurotransmitters dopamine and norepinephrine. An over-stimulation of the brain with the stimulatory neurotransmitters can deplete the brain of serotonin. I find it very difficult to balance serotonin levels in those that ingest aspartame. Aspartame should be avoided by everyone. Aspartame is the substance most reported to the FDA as having adverse effects.

THE CASE FOR DIAGNOSING AND TREATING FOOD ALLERGIES

My experience has clearly shown a relationship between food allergies and depression. Ingesting foods that are allergenic are very stressful for the body. Food allergies can manifest in a number of ways including runny nose and sneezing, headaches, asthma, hives and depression. Although any food allergy can precipitate depression, certain allergies seem to make the individual more prone to develop depression.

GLUTEN, SUGAR, AND DAIRY ALLERGIES

An allergy to gluten, the protein in wheat, is a common cause of depression. Approximately 1 in 133 people have celiac disease (an intestinal allergy to gluten) however, only 3% of people have currently been diagnosed in the U.S.[29] Gluten is found in other grains besides wheat, including rye, and barley. More information on a gluten-free diet can be found in my book, **_The Guide to a Gluten-Free Diet._**

Allergy to sugar is very common. My experience has shown that a sugar allergy can cause depression. An allergy to sugar can manifest as changes in blood sugar levels leading to hypoglycemic episodes. As previously mentioned, avoiding refined sugar is good dietary advice for everyone. As previously mentioned, artificial sweeteners such as Nutrasweet® and Splenda® should also be avoided.

Dairy allergies are also common with depression. I have seen countless patients improve many health conditions, including depression, by eliminating dairy from the diet. The pasteurization process of milk has altered the protein structure of milk and made it a very allergenic substance. Furthermore, the use of antibiotics and hormones in conventionally raised cattle has further exacerbated this condition. A simple blood test for casein antibodies can help diagnose this condition.   If you are going to ingest dairy products, I suggest you use dairy products from cows not fed antibiotics or hormones. More information on a dairy-free diet can be found in my book, ***The Guide to a Dairy-Free Diet.***

One way to effectively treat food allergies is to do an allergy elimination diet.   An allergy elimination diet consists of eliminating the offending food and observing the clinical results. Although an allergy elimination diet can seem daunting, it is a safe and effective way to help the body overcome illness.   A holistically-minded health care provider experienced with allergy elimination diets can help guide you. Keep in mind that it takes approximately six weeks for the body to fully adjust to being off an allergy provoking food. Therefore, you may have to wait up to six weeks to see if avoiding a particular food product will help your condition.

A simple, non toxic acupressure technique, NAET, has proven very useful to diagnose and treat food allergies. My 14 years of experience with NAET has shown its usefulness for treating food allergies. For more information on NAET, look at www.naet.com.

RAISING SEROTONIN LEVELS WITH LIGHT THERAPY

Exposure to adequate amounts of sunlight is a therapeutic way to increase your serotonin levels. In fact, researchers have shown that summer sunlight increases the brain serotonin levels twice as high as winter sunlight. Researchers concluded that, "...changes in {the} release of serotonin by the brain underlie mood seasonality and season affective disorder." [30] The light has to be of a certain intensity to be effective. Summer sunlight provides that intensity. In the Northern climates, fall and winter sunlight will not provide the intensity necessary to increase serotonin levels.

Seasonal affective disorder (SAD) affects a significant proportion of my patients. The low level of sunlight, resulting in lowered serotonin and Vitamin D levels that occurs in the fall and winter gives rise to SAD in those individuals that need adequate exposure to the sun. Those individuals with low serotonin levels will be dependant on exposure to adequate amounts of sunlight to stimulate serotonin production.

As previously mentioned, in the northern climates, it is the intensity of the sun which provides the body's needs for producing serotonin during the summer months. It is no surprise that I start hearing an increased frequency of depressive complaints from my patients in the fall and winter months.

Exposure to sunlamps (i.e., full spectrum lighting) can be helpful during the fall/winter months. Approximately 30-60 minutes per day, without sunglasses on can help. Full spectrum sun lamps can be purchased through NEEDS (800.634.1380). During the summer months, I counsel my patients to receive approximately 30 minutes of exposure to the sun, without sunscreen and sunglasses on.

In the fall/winter months Vitamin D supplementation has also proven helpful for those suffering from depression. This is particularly important for those residing in the northern climates. Vitamin D is known as the 'sunshine' vitamin. When high intensity sunlight hits the skin, a chemical reaction occurs whereby Vitamin D is produced from cholesterol. Vitamin D deficiency is rampant in the U.S. There are many reasons for this including the misguided information to avoid all sun exposure and the overuse of sunscreen preparations.

My experience has shown that some individuals are unable to raise their serotonin levels or their Vitamin D levels from supplementation alone. During the summer months exposure to the sun (approximately 15-30 minutes/day), without sunscreen, will usually solve the problem. During the winter months, tanning beds have also been helpful for some patients. In the winter months, the addition of 5-10 minutes in a tanning bed, three times per week, has proved sufficient to elevate the levels. More importantly, the use of tanning beds has improved depression in nearly all of these patients.

Many studies have shown the link between Vitamin D deficiency and depression.[31] [32] [33] [34] I recommend Vitamin D supplementation to most of my patients during the winter months (from 1,000U to 10,000U/day). However, Vitamin D supplementation can be toxic. Although I have rarely seen problems with Vitamin D supplementation, I suggest that you consult with your nutritionally oriented health care provider to periodically check Vitamin D levels. Vitamin D toxicity can be avoided by appropriately supplementing the other fat soluble vitamins including Vitamins A, E and K.

CAN HORMONE IMBALANCES CAUSE DEPRESSION?

The answer to the above question is unequivocally, yes. The relationship between hormone imbalances and depression has been discussed in the medical literature for over 100 years. Hormones control all physiologic processes in the body. Adequate hormone production is necessary for balancing our mood as well as maintaining a healthy immune system. The underlying cause of many chronic illnesses, including depression may be a hormonal imbalance.

Depression is often a symptom of an imbalanced hormonal system. Most frequently, I see thyroid and adrenal imbalances leading to depression. In these cases, treatment with an antidepressant will only target the symptom—depression—and not the underlying cause—the thyroid and/or adrenal imbalance.

I have seen numerous patients given the label of depression and treated with an antidepressant who have never had a thorough evaluation of their hormonal system. When the underlying imbalanced hormonal system is corrected with the use of bioidentical natural hormones, with great frequency, depression and other mood disorders either significantly improve or resolve. It is rare not to see improvement in depression when the hormonal system is properly rebalanced.

Tracy is a 34 year-old female who was well until she got pregnant with her third child. Tracy became very fatigued during the pregnancy and gained a tremendous amount of weight—75 pounds. After the birth of her child, Tracy was fatigued and depressed. "I couldn't lose the weight I had gained during the pregnancy. I was also exhausted--much more so than just having a baby. My doctor kept telling me it was normal, with my busy household, but I knew better," she said. Tracy's doctor referred her to a psychiatrist and told her she was depressed. Tracy commented, "I knew I was depressed. But, I was depressed because I felt so bad, not the other way around." When I took a thorough history from Tracy, she had many signs and symptoms of hypothyroidism, including being fatigued, feeling cold, having cold hands and feet, constipation, and hair loss. She also had a very low basal body temperature—96.4 degrees Fahrenheit (normal 97.8-98.2 degrees Fahrenheit). Tracy's blood tests revealed a hypothyroid condition. When I explained to her that I thought her thyroid condition was responsible for how she was feeling she began to cry. "I was so happy for someone to tell me that I am not crazy. I knew there had to be a reason I was feeling this way," she said. I also found that Tracy had multiple hormonal imbalances including low progesterone and DHEA levels. Tracy was treated with desiccated thyroid (Armour®thyroid), natural progesterone and DHEA along with a holistic nutritional program. Within four weeks she was feeling markedly better, having no signs of depression. Tracy claimed, "It was truly miraculous. My brain came back on-line. I actually felt back to myself. This has given me my life back."

Tracy's case is not uncommon. The relationship between hypothyroidism and depression has been known for over 100 years. For more information on thyroid disorders, I refer the reader to ***Overcoming Thyroid Disorders, 2nd Edition***.

Doctors are all too quick to prescribe an antidepressant medication without exploring all options. No patient has an 'antidepressant medication deficiency'. There are many causes of depression. A thorough history and physical exam needs to be performed before prescribing and taking an antidepressant. Common sense would dictate that the underlying cause of depression needs to be thoroughly searched for. When treating depression, an antidepressant medication should be the last resort, not the first resort.

IS THERE A BENEFIT TO ANTIDEPRESSANT DRUG THERAPY?

Yes. The antidepressant drugs do work in some people and can have miraculous effects. However, their benefits are overstated by Big Pharma. In cases of mild to moderate depression, I believe that drug therapies should be a last resort. Oftentimes, antidepressant drug therapies result in a patient becoming dependant on the drug. It can be very difficult to come off these medications.

As previously mentioned, drug therapies disrupt the normal brain function by poisoning a crucial enzyme. Furthermore, the long-term use of a drug therapy often leads to a dependency on that drug. Generally, the longer a drug is used, the more adverse effects will occur.

In cases of serious depression, a short course of a drug therapy may be warranted. However, a drug therapy should be combined with either psychotherapy or another non-drug therapy such as exercise. These non-drug therapies will enable the patient to use a lowered amount of the drug and use the drug for a shorter course.

Drug therapies may have a faster onset of action as compared to non-drug therapies such as psychotherapy. In a case of serious depression, drug therapies may be an appropriate first-

236

line choice. However, all drug therapies can be improved with a more holistic approach which emphasizes diet and nutrition.

FINAL THOUGHTS: PUTTING IT ALL TOGETHOR

Antidepressant medications are some of the most commonly prescribed medications. At the first sign of depression, doctors are too quick to write a prescription for an antidepressant medication.

Depression is a debilitating illness. In most cases, depression can be effectively managed with non-drug therapies. The first step for any depressed patient is to examine the food they are eating. Improving the diet by eliminating refined foods is the first step to take. I have seen countless patients overcome depression simply by changing their diet. For more information on how to implement a healthier diet, I refer the reader to my book, ***The Guide to Healthy Eating.***

For the majority of people with depression, antidepressant drugs should be used as a last resort. There are many safe and effective non-drug therapies that can be used first such as psychotherapy and exercise.

[1] Vedantam, S. Washington Post. Dec. 3, 2004. p. A15

[2] http://www.nimh.hih.gov/publicat/numbers.cfm. Accessed 5.13.06

[3] http://www.nimh.hih.gov/publicat/numbers.cfm. Accessed 5.13.06

[4] http://www.pharmacytimes.com/article.cfm?ID=2534. Accessed 5.13.06

[5] Hart, Carol. Secrets of Serotonin. St. Martin's Press. 1996

[6] The Columbia Encyclopedia, Sixth Edition 2006

[7] Hart, Carol. IBID.

[8] Sernbach, H. The Serotonin Syndrome. Am. J. of Psych. 148:6, 705-13. June, 1991.

[9] Khan, A. Symptom reduction and suicide risk in patients treated with placebo in antidepressant clinical trials: An Analysis of the food and Drug Administration Database. Arch. Of Gen. Psychiatry. 57:311-17. 2000

[10] Breggin, Peter. The Anti-Depressant Fact Book. Perseus Publ. 2001. Reprinted by permission of Da Capo Press, a member of Perseus Books Group

[11] Watkins, L. Anitidepressant use in coronary heart disease patients: Impact on survival. Presented at 64th Annual Scientific Conference of the American Psychosomatic Society in Denver, March 4, 2006

[12] Rowan, R. Second Opinion Newsletter. July, 2006

[13] N. Eng. J. of Med. 2006;354:579-87

[14] FDA Talk Paper. July 1, 2005

[15] Arch. of Gen. Psychiatry. August 2006;63(8):865-872

[16] J. Am. Acad. Child Psychiatry. 2003;42:22-29

[17] JAMA. Feb. 23, 2000;283:1025-30

[18] FP News. 9.15.06

[19] Glenmullen, G. Prozac Backlash. Simon and Shuster. 2000.

[20] Elkin, I. National Institute of Mental Health treatment of depression collaborative research program: general effectiveness of treatments. Arch.of Gen. Psych. 46(1989):971-82

[21] British J. of Psych. 139. 1981: 181-9

[22] Cognitive Therapy and Research. 1. 1977, 17-37

[23] Am. J. of Psych. 136 (1979): 555-58.

[24] Am. J. of Psych. 148 (1991) 784-89

[25] Arch. of Gen. Psych. 56 1999, 431-37

[26] J. of Consulting and Clin. Psych. 61(1993); 858-64

[27] Prusoff, A. Differential symptom reduction by drugs and psychotherapy in acute depression. Arch. of Gen. Psych. 36 (1979): 1450-56

[28] Babyak, M. Exercise treatment for major depression: maintenance of therapeutic benefit at 10 months. Psychosomatic Medicine. 62:633-638. 2000

[29] Fasano, A. Arch. of Int. Med. 2003;163:286-92

[30] Lambert, GW. Effect of sunlight and season on serotonin turnover in the brain. Lancet. 2002. Dec. 7;360(9348): 1840-2

[31] Stumpf, W. Light, vitamin D and psychiatry. Role of 1,25 dihydroxyvitamn D3 in etiology and therapy of seasonal affective disorder and other mental processes. Psychopharmacology (Berl). 1989;97(3):285-94

[32] Landsdown, A. Vitamin D3 enhances mood in healthy subjects during winter. Psychopharmacology (Berl). 1998 Feb;135(4):319-23

33 Gloth, FM. Vitamin D vs broad spectrum phototherapy in the treatment of seasonal affective disorder. J. Nutr. Health Aging. 1999;3(1):5-7

34 Schneider, B. Vitamin D in schizophrenia, major depression and alcoholism. J Neural Transm. 2000;107(7):839-42.

Chapter 8

Anti-inflammatory Drugs

INTRODUCTION

Anti-inflammatory medications are some of the most commonly prescribed drugs. More than 100 million prescriptions for NSAID's are written annually in the United States.[1] It is estimated that more than 30 million people worldwide take anti-inflammatory medications on a daily basis.[2] This number does not include the over-the-counter use of NSAID's such as aspirin and Motrin®. Examples of anti-inflammatory medications are shown in Table 1. These medications are often referred to as 'non-steroidal anti-inflammatory drugs' (NSAID's).

TABLE 1: EXAMPLES OF ANTI-INFLAMMATORY MEDICATIONS

Aspirin
Celcoxib   (Celebrex®)
Diclofenac   (Voltaren®)
Ibuprofen   (Motrin®)
Indomethacin (Indocin®)
Ketoprofen   (Orudis®)
Naproxen   (Naprosyn®)
Piroxicam   (Feldene®)
Rofecoxib   (Vioxx®)

NSAID'S AND PROSTAGLANDINS

What are NSAID's? NSAID's are a class of medications that poison an enzyme in the prostaglandin pathway. Prostaglandins are a group of hormone-like substances present in many body tissues and body fluids. Prostaglandins regulate many important bodily functions including clotting of the blood and protecting the stomach lining from acid. In addition, prostaglandins control inflammation, fever, and pain in the body. Prostaglandins play a vital role in most physiologic processes of the body. Table 2 lists many of the vital processes that prostaglandins regulate.

TABLE 2: EXAMPLES OF PHYSIOLOGIC PROCESSES THAT PROSTAGLANDINS REGULATE

Bone formation	Hemostasis (blood clotting)
Bone resorption	Mucosal integrity of the GI tract
Bronchial tone	Immune function
Central nervous system functioning	Ovulation
Digestion	Parturition
Febrile response	Pain sensation
Fertilization	Platelet aggregation
Fetal development	Renal blood flow

Prostaglandins have been implicated in a number of disease states that have an inflammatory component such as asthma, arthritis, and inflammatory bowel disorders such as colitis. Furthermore, prostaglandins have been associated with cancer and Alzheimer's disease. Due to the large number of disease processes that prostaglandins affect, there has been a lot of interest in developing drugs that affect prostaglandins.

HOW DO NSAID's AFFECT PROSTAGLANDINS?

NSAID's affect prostaglandin synthesis by poisoning an enzyme (cyclooxygenase) that is responsible for facilitating the production of prostaglandins. There are two major classes of enzymes that NSAID's affect in the body and they are known as cyclooxygenase-1 (Cox-1) and cyclooxygenase-2 (Cox-2). These enzymes facilitate the conversion of the fatty acid arachidonic acid into many different prostaglandins. This pathway is shown in Figure 1 (page 244).

The pathway begins from the unsaturated fatty acid, arachidonic acid. Arachidonic acid is obtained from the diet either from animal fats or it is synthesized in the body. Too much arachidonic acid has been thought to provide fuel for the body's over-production of inflammatory prostaglandins.

As discussed in ***The Guide to Healthy Eating,*** the Standard American Diet provides far too many poor quality Omega-6 fatty acids and thus an overabundance of arachidonic acid. Omega-6 fatty acids are found in a variety of foods such as animal products as well as refined vegetable oils (e.g., corn, safflower, and canola). Increasing the consumption of Omega-3 fatty acids (found in fish, fish oil, flaxseed oil and walnuts) can help reduce arachidonic acid and help lower the amount of pro-inflammatory prostaglandins.

Later in this chapter you will find a section on fish oil and other ways to increase Omega-3 fatty acids.

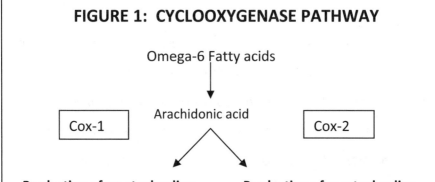

FIGURE 1: CYCLOOXYGENASE PATHWAY

Omega-6 Fatty acids

Arachidonic acid

Cox-1

Cox-2

Production of prostaglandins (thromboxane) responsible for:
- Platelet activation
- Stomach protection
- Kidney function
- Increase smooth muscle cell proliferation
- Vasoconstriction

Production of prostaglandins (Prostaglandin E2) responsible for:
- Inflammation

Production of Prostaglandins (Prostacyclin) responsible for:
- Inhibit platelet aggregation
- Induce arterial dilation
- Prevent proliferation of smooth muscle cells in the artery walls

As can be seen from Figure 1, the Cox-1 enzyme produces prostaglandins which are responsible for many different functions in the body including platelet activation, stomach protection, and kidney function. In contrast, the Cox-2 enzyme is responsible for the production of prostaglandins (prostaglandin E2) which control the inflammatory response. However, the Cox-2 enzyme also helps produce other prostaglandins (e.g., prostacyclin) which prevent blood clots by;

1. Inhibiting platelet aggregation
2. Inducing arterial dilation
3. Preventing the proliferation of smooth muscle cells in the arterial walls

Since the Cox-2 enzyme has multiple contrasting effects, the effects of poisoning that enzyme cannot be predicted in the individual patient. Perhaps, in some, a Cox-2 blocker medication will have an anti-inflammatory effect. However, in others, a Cox-2 blocker medication may increase the risk of blood clots—such as strokes and heart attacks.

Most of the older, traditional NSAID's such as Motrin® and aspirin block the functioning of Cox-1 and have a lowered (or little) ability to block the Cox-2 enzyme. The newer NSAID's, Vioxx® and Celebrex® are more specific in inhibiting the Cox-2 enzyme.

WHAT ARE NSAID'S USED FOR?

As mentioned previously, NSAID's are some of the most commonly prescribed medications in the United States. They account for a multi-billion dollar stream of revenue for Big Pharma. NSAID's are used to treat inflammation in the body. The inflammatory response in the body can take many different forms including pain, swelling, redness, warmth, and fever.

Everybody has experienced inflammation in their body. If you sprain your ankle, the swelling, warmth, and redness around the injured ankle are all signs of the inflammatory response. The inflammatory response of the body is a normal physiologic response. In the sprained ankle example, the swelling occurs due to fluid leaking out of injured capillaries in the ligament that has been strained. This fluid contains prostaglandins which promote inflammation and swelling. The swelling distends the tissue which compresses nerves and causes pain.

The warmth of the injured tissues helps to prevent an infection. The prostaglandins help to recruit white blood cells to the injured area. The white blood cells help to prevent an infection as well as clear up cellular debris. Other chemicals are released by the body to increase the release of certain white blood cells and immune system cells which all aid in the healing process.

Although none of us enjoys inflammation (and the resulting pain and swelling) that accompanies an injury, the inflammation serves a number of purposes. It helps to recruit certain immune system cells that promote the healing of the injured tissue. Furthermore, inflammation sends a message (i.e., pain) that the injured area needs to rest. Further use of an already injured body part may lead to worsening the injury. The inflammation is the body's way of telling us to rest so that it can heal itself. There are many triggers that promote inflammation. Table 3 gives examples of these inflammatory triggers.[3]

Table 3: Triggers of Inflammation
Bacteria
Cell-wall debris
Drugs
Environmental toxins
Food antigens
Free radical damage
Fungi
Injury
Leaky gut
Parasites
Suppression of anti-inflammatory prostaglandin synthesis
Trauma
Viruses
Yeast

Of all the conditions listed in Table 3, which ones do NSAID's treat? NSAID's do not treat any of them. In fact, their long-term use will make many of these triggers worse. Conventional medicine recommends prescribing a NSAID for nearly all inflammatory conditions. I think a better approach is to look for the underlying cause of inflammation. Then, the appropriate therapy to treat the underlying cause can be prescribed.   Identifying and treating the root cause of inflammation should be the goal. This comprehensive and holistic approach will lead to a better outcome as compared to just prescribing a NSAID.

NSAID's block the inflammatory response by poisoning the COX enzymes (see Figure 1, page 244). Although NSAID's may help with symptom relief, they do little to promote healing. In fact, their long-term use will actually inhibit healing. Keep in mind, in the case of an ankle sprain, the underlying problem is the strained ligament. The swelling and pain are only the symptoms of the underlying problem. Taking an anti-inflammatory medication does little to help the underlying problem of ligament strain. In fact, the long-term use of an anti-inflammatory medication will inhibit healing of the sprain. Remember, anti-inflammatory medications only treat the symptoms of the injury.

Our body is a wonderful machine. When a piece of the machine is broken, it needs to be repaired. If we give our body the correct raw materials (vitamins, minerals, enzymes, water, etc.), complete healing will often occur. In the example of the sprained ankle, the body needs adequate amounts of Vitamin C to help promote collagen formation and repair the injured ankle ligament. Inadequate body stores of Vitamin C will lead to a poor outcome.

Inflammation is not a sign of an 'NSAID deficiency'. Inflammation is a normal response of the body to an injury. The inflammatory response of the body can be treated with nutritional support which supplies the body with the correct agents to allow it to heal the injury. Later in this chapter we will discuss which nutrients help in the healing process.

WHAT IS THE DIFFERENCE BETWEEN OLDER AND NEWER (COX-2) NSAID'S?

All of the NSAID's reduce the inflammatory response in the body by inhibiting the cyclooxygenase enzyme (Cox-1 and Cox-2). As previously mentioned, the older NSAID's, such as Motrin®, aspirin, and Naprosyn®, generally are more specific for inhibiting the Cox-1 enzyme.

As can be seen from Figure 1, the poisoning of the Cox-1 enzyme inhibits the production of certain prostaglandins (thromboxane) that mediate many important physiologic functions in the body including the production of mucous that protects the gastrointestinal tract. This inhibition will leave the stomach vulnerable for ulcerations. This is why the long-term use of all the NSAID's (e.g., aspirin or Motrin®) are associated with gastrointestinal bleeding and ulcerations. In fact, a recent study of over 88,000 subjects found the risk of gastrointestinal ulcerations and bleeding increased by 212% with Naprosyn® and 96% with Voltarin®.

Cox-2 inhibitors were advertised as having fewer side effects than the older Cox-1 inhibitors. This class of medications includes Vioxx® and Celebrex®. Big Pharma promoted these agents as much safer than the older NSAID's since they do not inhibit the Cox-1 enzyme.

COX-2 INHIBITORS: VIOXX®
AND CELEBREX®

In 1999, Vioxx® and Celebrex® were the first two Cox-2 inhibitors approved by the FDA for treating arthritic symptoms. Big Pharma went on a major advertising blitz, telling doctors and the public that there would be fewer side effects, especially gastrointestinal side effects. From 2000 to 2001, Celebrex sales totaled $2.3 billion and Vioxx® sales totaled $1.7 billion. Clever advertising and marketing certainly worked for these pharmaceuticals; they instantly became blockbuster drugs.

Were there fewer side effects with the Cox-2's as compared to the older NSAID's such as aspirin and Motrin®? Did patients save money switching to the new class of NSAID's that Big Pharma was promoting?

The answer to both of the above questions is a resounding "No".

DO THE COX-2 NSAID'S OFFER PROTECTION AGAINST GASTROINTESTINAL BLEEDING AS COMPARED TO THE OLDER NSAID'S?

Since their initial use in the 1950's, NSAID's have been associated with significant morbidity and mortality. This is primarily due to the gastrointestinal adverse effects of ulceration and bleeding.[4] In fact, over 100,000 hospitalizations occur annually in the United States due to gastrointestinal adverse effects due to NSAID's.[5] Estimates are that up to 4.5% of NSAID users can develop serious gastrointestinal events including ulcers and bleeding.[6][7][8] There is a 400% increased risk in hospitalization with NSAID use.[9] During my residency, I saw countless patients admitted to the hospital for gastrointestinal bleeding secondary to NSAID use.

Big-Pharma promoted Cox-2 inhibitors (Vioxx® and Celebrex®) as being safer than traditional NSAID's due to Cox-2 inhibitors having less gastrointestinal toxicity. The ads were very appealing to doctors. Who wouldn't want to prescribe a safer NSAID?

Were the Cox-2 inhibitors safer than the older NSAID's? Unfortunately, the research never showed that Cox-2 inhibitors offered a safer alternative as compared to the older NSAID's. In fact, the initial research pointed out potentially serious problems with the Cox-2 inhibitors. Follow up studies confirmed the problems with the Cox-2 inhibitors. This information certainly was not found in the advertising materials that Big Pharma was promoting.

A study comparing Vioxx® to placebo found the risk of serious gastrointestinal side effects was five times greater in those that took Vioxx®.[10] This 5-fold increase in gastrointestinal

251

side effects is similar (or even higher) to the rate found for all NSAID's. Another study of Celebrex® (Cox-2 inhibitor) found that there was no difference in the rate of gastrointestinal bleeding between Celebrex® and diclofenac (Voltarin®--an older NSAID).[11] Another study of 8,059 arthritic patients found that Celebrex® offered no gastrointestinal benefit over ibuprofen (Motrin®) or diclofenac (Feldene®--an older NSAID).[12]

Big Pharma ran ads in the medical journals, on television, and in the print media claiming that Cox-2 inhibitors would have less gastrointestinal side effects as compared to older NSAID's. However, the research never proved this claim. In fact, the research indicated there was no substantial difference on the effect of gastrointestinal bleeding between the newer and older NSAID's. Yet, through direct-to-consumer advertising and clever marketing techniques, Cox-2 agents became blockbuster drugs for Big Pharma. However, the wide-spread prescribing of Cox-2 inhibitors was leading to more serious adverse effects.

DO COX-2 INHIBITORS LEAD TO MORE CARDIOVASCULAR DEATHS?

Who has not seen the headlines in the newspapers or seen the news stories about all the cardiovascular deaths associated with Vioxx®? The pharmaceutical company, Merck & Co., Inc., is embroiled in thousands of lawsuits alleging Vioxx was responsible for nearly 50,000 deaths and 150,000 strokes and heart attacks.

Was the stroke/heart attack risk for Cox-2 inhibitors predictable? The answer to this question is "Yes". Let's review the mechanism of action of the Cox-2 inhibitors.

THE YIN AND YANG OF COX-1 AND COX-2 ENZYMES

Our bodies have multiple checks and balances. The Chinese refer to this as the 'Yin and Yang'. For example, we have a parasympathetic and a sympathetic nervous system, both working to maintain homeostasis in the body. The sympathetic nervous system helps us with the 'fight or flight' response. The parasympathetic nervous system does the opposite by helping us 'rest and digest'. Our body strives to achieve a proper balance between the parasympathetic and the sympathetic nervous system. The body does not want one system to dominate the other. Chronic illness and poor health will be the outcome if there is an imbalance between the parasympathetic and sympathetic nervous systems.

Although Cox-1 and Cox-2 pathways are not strictly opposites of one another, the body strives to maintain a balance between the two pathways. An overactive Cox-2 pathway tends to promote inflammation. An overactive Cox-1 pathway may lead to blood clots, strokes and heart attacks. When good health is present, there is a balance between the Cox-1 and the Cox-2 pathways. If we look at Figure 1 (page 244), selectively poisoning the Cox-2 enzyme may (theoretically) result in less inflammation by decreasing the production of the inflammatory prostaglandin E2. However other prostaglandins, such as prostacyclin, are also dependant on the Cox-2 enzyme. Prostacyclin is responsible for inhibiting platelet aggregation (clotting), helping the blood vessels dilate, and preventing the proliferation of smooth muscle cells in the arterial wall.[13] [14] All of these functions help decrease the risk of blood clotting disorders such as stroke and heart attacks.

Furthermore, if the Cox-2 enzyme is poisoned, that leaves the Cox-1 enzyme unopposed. Now, the yin/yang balance of the Cox-1 and Cox-2 enzymes is upset. An unopposed Cox-1 pathway may lead to platelet aggregation (clotting) and blood vessel constriction--two conditions that can lead to an increased incidence of strokes and heart attacks. Some scientists that initially looked at the mechanism of action of the Cox-2 inhibitors predicted an increased risk of blood-clotting disorders such as stroke and heart attacks in patients that would take a Cox-2 inhibitor.

Our bodies need balance. There are not good and bad Cox enzymes. There are no good and bad prostaglandins. Inflammation is not bad for our bodies. Our bodies require a balance between anti-inflammatory prostaglandins and pro-inflammatory prostaglandins. When we give our bodies the raw materials (vitamins, minerals, enzymes, etc.) they need, our bodies can maintain homeostasis and take care of themselves.

What is the end-result of poisoning the Cox-2 enzyme? So far, at least 50,000 deaths and 150,000 strokes and heart attacks are adverse effects attributed to the Cox-2 inhibitors. *Remember, poisoning a crucial enzyme or blocking an important receptor for the long-term is a recipe for a poor outcome.*

DO NSAID'S ADVERSELY AFFECT THE KIDNEYS?

Long-term NSAID use is known to adversely affect kidney function. It is estimated that over 2.5 million individuals in the United States experience adverse renal effects caused by the use of NSAID's.[15] NSAID's have been proven to adversely affect kidney function by: [16] [17] [18]

1. Decreasing renal perfusion

2. Decreasing glomerular filtration rate

3. Causing edema

4. Increasing blood pressure

5. Causing interstitial nephritis

Cox-2 inhibitors were initially promoted by Big Pharma as being significantly safer for the kidneys as compared to older NSAID's--this was part of the marketing message sent to doctors about these medications.

However, researchers found that Cox-2 inhibitors can

negatively affect kidney function at the same rate as the older NSAID's. In 2000, researchers reported that both the old (Indocin®) and the new Cox-2 NSAID (Vioxx®) significantly decreased the kidney's ability to filter out waste products.[19] Furthermore, researchers pointed out that the patients who are at an increased risk of kidney dysfunction from NSAID use are those who are on a salt-restricted diet, diuretic therapy, or those who have reduced kidney function, hypertension, congestive heart failure, or liver disease.

Decreased kidney function can result in an excess accumulation of homocysteine and a marked increase in mortality from heart attacks and strokes. More on this topic will be found later in this chapter.

DOES CELEBREX® HAVE A LOWERED RISK AS COMPARED TO VIOXX®?

The answer appears to be "Yes". Celebrex® is less Cox-2 selective than Vioxx®. Again, looking at the pathway for the Cox-2 enzyme (Figure 1), a less selective inhibitor of this enzyme would lead one to conclude that it will have less serious adverse cardiovascular events as compared to a more specific Cox-2 inhibitor (such as Vioxx®). However, even if Celebrex® does not poison the Cox-2 pathway quite as much as Vioxx®, it still has a significant inhibitory effect on the Cox-2 enzyme. Whenever you inhibit the Cox-2 enzyme and disrupt the balance between the

Cox-1 and Cox-2 systems, you will increase the risk of adverse effects such as platelet aggregation (blood clots), and vasoconstriction.

There has been little data that supports the idea that Cox-2 inhibitors provide more gastrointestinal protection as compared to older NSAID's. So why did the Cox-2 inhibitors become so widely prescribed? Clever advertising and marketing certainly can sell a lot of drugs.

DO OTHER NSAID'S CAUSE AN INCREASE IN HEART ATTACKS?

Even older NSAID's have many adverse effects associated with their use. As was previously discussed, the most common adverse effect of NSAID's is gastrointestinal (G.I.) bleeding. G.I. bleeding occurs because the production of prostaglandins which protect the stomach lining is being impeded by taking the NSAID. However, some of the older, widely used NSAID's have also been associated with an increase in heart attacks.

A recent study in the British Medical Journal found several NSAID's associated with an increased risk of heart attacks. The following medications were found to increase the risk of heart attacks:[20]

    1. Voltaren® (55% increase)

    2. Ibuprofen (24% increase)

    3. Naprosyn (32% increase)

Why would the older NSAID's also increase the heart attack risk? All NSAID's have some capabilities to poison both Cox-1 and Cox-2 enzymes. *Keep in mind that you cannot poison a crucial enzyme or block an important receptor for the long-term and expect a good result.* By poisoning enzymes in the Cox pathways, adverse effects are bound to be present.

Another reason for NSAID's causing heart disease has to do with NSAID's decreasing the blood flow to the kidneys. NSAID's have been shown to cause kidney failure.[21] [22] [23] Kidney disease has been associated with a high rate of cardiovascular disease as well as high homocysteine levels. Researchers feel that high homocysteine levels, which are present in severe kidney failure, are a major reason for the high cardiovascular mortality rate.[24] [25]

WHAT WERE THE CONSEQUENCES OF HYPING THE COX-2 MEDICATIONS?

As previously mentioned, the Cox-2 inhibitors offered no substantial benefit in reducing the risk of gastrointestinal side effects as compared to older NSAID drugs. By poisoning the Cox-2 enzyme, the Cox-2 inhibitors have been shown to increase the risk of stroke and heart attacks as well as increase the risk of death. Vioxx® was approved in 1999. By 2003, Vioxx® accounted for $2.5 billion in worldwide sales. The first study that showed there may be an increased risk of stroke and heart attacks appeared shortly after Vioxx® was released in 2000.[26] Estimates are that over

140,000 Americans suffered serious adverse effects and nearly 50,000 died due to Vioxx®. Vioxx® was not pulled from the market until 2004. How could this happen and why didn't the FDA act sooner?

WHY DID IT TAKE SO LONG FOR VIOXX® TO BE PULLED FROM THE MARKET?

As mentioned above, the first reports of adverse effects from Vioxx® appeared shortly after it was approved in 2000. The VIGOR study found that there was a significantly increased risk of heart attacks and strokes in those subjects that took Vioxx®.[27] By the time Vioxx® was withdrawn four years later, over 80 million people had taken it and there were reports of numerous deaths and heart attacks associated with its use.[28]

There is much blame to go around for the Vioxx® debacle. It is an example of "masterful public relations, aggressive marketing and ineffective regulation."[29] Dr. Eric Topol, chief of cardiovascular medicine at Cleveland Clinic said, "The FDA didn't do anything. They were ineffective."[30]

One courageous man, Dr. David Graham, a 20-year FDA drug researcher, tried to expose the information about Vioxx®. He reported that in the United States, approximately 140,000 cardiovascular events (stroke and/or heart attack) occurred and 50,000 people died since Vioxx® was approved.[31] Dr. Graham testified before a Senate subcommittee on his findings. He called the FDA's oversight of Vioxx® "a profound regulatory failure".[32] Due to his testimony, Dr. Graham was intimidated by his FDA supervisors and retaliated against. Dr. Graham has stated, "As currently configured, the FDA is not able to adequately protect the American public. It is more interested in protecting the interest of industry."[33]

I believe if physicians had studied the mechanisms for how the Cox-2 inhibitors affected the body, they would have been wary about their wide-spread use. *Remember, you can't poison a crucial enzyme or block an important receptor and expect a good long-term result.*

ADVERSE EFFECTS OF NSAID'S

As with most medications that poison enzymes or block receptors, there are multiple adverse effects of NSAID's. Table 4 lists some of these adverse effects.

TABLE 4: ADVERSE EFFECTS OF NSAIDS	
Bleeding	Kidney failure
Constipation	Leaky gut
Decreased appetite	Liver failure
Depression	Nausea
Diarrhea	Poor healing
Dizziness	Rash
Drowsiness	Reduce blood flow to kidneys
Edema	Reduce action of diuretics
Fluid retention	Shortness of breath
Gastrointestinal bleeding	Sleep disturbance
Headache	Ulcers
Increased risk of heart attack	Vomiting

NSAID's have been shown to increase gut permeability which can allow toxins to enter the circulatory system.[34] This can lead to leaky gut syndrome which is common with long-term NSAID use.

In 1994, Lester Crawford, the FDA commissioner claimed, "All the NSAID drugs have risks when taken chronically, especially of gastrointestinal bleeding, but also of liver and kidney toxicity. They should only be used continuously under the supervision of a physician."[35]

SHOULD NSAID'S EVER BE USED?

All drugs have their time and place. However, I feel any drug that poisons a crucial enzyme or blocks an important receptor should be used only with extreme caution. Furthermore, drugs that poison enzymes and block receptors should be used for the shortest term possible. There are occasions when these drugs need to be used for the long-term. However, the long-term use of these medications should be a last resort.

NSAID's are very good drugs for short-term use. In the case of an ankle sprain, NSAID's can be effective at lowering the pain associated with the sprain. However, they should not be used for the long-term. There are many safe and effective anti-inflammatory therapies that can be used for the long-term.

These natural alternatives to NSAID's have far fewer side effects and are much safer for the body (see Table 5, page 263).

Furthermore, the addition of natural anti-inflammatory agents can both lower the amount of NSAID's needed and also decrease the length of time they are required.

Cox-2 inhibitors cause many more serious adverse effects as compared to older NSAID's. If an NSAID is needed, I would recommend staying with a time-tested older NSAID as opposed to a newer version. Ibuprofen has a long track record. Although it does have adverse effects such as increasing the risk of gastrointestinal bleeding, it is inexpensive and does not have the serious cardiovascular adverse effects the Cox-2 inhibitors have. Ibuprofen should be considered as a first-line agent when a NSAID is going to be prescribed.

NATURAL ANTI-INFLAMMATORY ALTERNATIVES

There are many safe and effective natural anti-inflammatory options available. My experience has shown that these natural alternatives can often be as effective--sometimes more effective--as compared to any NSAID. These natural alternatives have a much lowered risk of an adverse effect. Table 5 gives some examples of natural anti-inflammatory agents.

TABLE 5: EXAMPLES OF NATURAL ANTI-INFLAMMATORY AGENTS

Black currant oil	Glucosamine
Borage oil	Green tea
Boswellic extract	Hops
Cherry juice	Hyaluronic acid
Curcumin	Lipoic acid
Digestive enzymes	Maintaining adequate hydration
Evening primrose oil	Methylsulfonylmethane (MSM)
Fish oil	Serrapeptase
Flavinoids	Tumeric
Flaxseed oil	Vitamin C

Fish Oil

Your diet can have a profound effect on whether you will be more prone to developing an inflammatory condition such as arthritis. An unhealthy diet will be pro-inflammatory. A healthy diet will not only be anti-inflammatory, it will promote a healthy immune and hormonal system. Eating food that contains refined oils (as well as refined carbohydrates) will be pro-inflammatory. Eating healthy food containing unrefined oils will be anti-inflammatory.

There are good fats and bad fats. Fats provide fatty acids for the body. Life is not possible without adequate amounts of good fatty acids. Good fats contain substances the body can use to maintain structure and produce energy. Good fats are essential to maintain a healthy immune and hormonal system.

Bad fats not only provide no nutrition to the body, they also cause the immune system to malfunction and can lead to a variety of inflammatory illnesses such as obesity, cancer, and autoimmune problems. Ingesting the right form of fatty acids can have a powerful anti-inflammatory effect in the body. Conversely, ingesting the wrong form of fatty acids can have a marked pro-inflammatory effect.

Eating the correct balance of Omega-6 and Omega-3 fatty acids (approximately a 4:1 Omega-6/Omega-3) provides the body with the essential fatty acids necessary to reduce inflammation. The Standard American Diet contains too many Omega-6 fatty acids and too little Omega-3 fatty acids. Estimates are that the Standard American Diet contains approximately a 20-40:1 ratio of Omega-6 fatty acids to Omega-3 fatty acids. This high ratio of Omega-6 fatty acids leads to inflammatory disorders, obesity, cancer, and autoimmune disorders as well as a whole host of chronic illnesses.

Processed vegetable oils (i.e., refined vegetable oils) are the most common culprits in disrupting the Omega-6:Omega-3 ratio. These oils contain high amounts of poor-quality Omega-6 fats without the balancing effect of Omega-3 fats. Many of these oils (soybean, canola, corn, and cottonseed) contain harmful free radicals due to their processing techniques. An unhealthy balance of Omega-6 fatty acids is found in many common supermarket foods such as non-organic eggs, farm-raised fish, and conventionally raised meat, as well as refined vegetable oils. Furthermore, cookies, cakes, crackers, etc., that have been made with these refined oils will contain unhealthy fatty acids. Due to the prevalence of food items that contain these refined oils, is it any wonder that inflammatory conditions such as arthritis are skyrocketing today?

Refined oils, like all refined food, needs to be avoided. For more information about oils, I refer the reader to ***The Guide to Healthy Eating.***

Decreasing the intake of refined fats and increasing the amount of Omega-3 fats in the diet can have a profound anti-inflammatory effect on the body. Fish oil contains the anti-inflammatory fatty acids, EPA and DHA. These agents have been found to reduce inflammatory prostaglandins (Prostaglandin E-2 and Leukotrien B-4).[36] Good sources of EPA and DHA include cold-water fish such as wild salmon, as well as cod and cod liver oil. Fish oil can be a helpful source for obtaining Omega-3 fats. Fish oil has been found to significantly reduce pain and stiffness in osteoarthritis.[37] There are numerous studies showing the anti-inflammatory benefits of Omega-3 fatty acids for rheumatoid arthritis sufferers.[38 39 40] Omega-3 fatty acids have been shown to help improve stiffness and grip strength. Their use has also been found to decrease swelling in joints and lower the pain index in arthritis.

RECOMMENDATIONS FOR FATTY ACIDS

Avoid refined vegetable oils such as soybean, canola, corn, and cottonseed. Use healthy cooking oils such as coconut and olive oil. Omega-3 oils cannot be used for cooking; they should not be heated. I suggest that you eat cold-water fish at least two times per week or take fish oil capsules, 3gm/day (generally three capsules/day). However, this must be accompanied with improving your diet and eliminating or decreasing the amount of refined Omega-6 oils in your diet. Much more dietary information can be found in ***The Guide to Healthy Eating.***

GLUCOSAMINE

Glucosamine and chondroitin sulfate are substances found naturally in the body. Glucosamine is a sugar that provides the ground substance that forms cartilage. Studies have shown that glucosamine has been found to benefit patients with arthritis.[41] My experience has shown that many patients with arthritic symptoms improve with glucosamine. Unlike NSAID's, there are little side effects with glucosamine. **RECOMMENDATIONS:** Try 500mg of glucosamine three times per day for six weeks. If you don't see a response in six weeks, discontinue it.

SYSTEMIC ENZYMES

Systemic enzymes have very potent anti-inflammatory effects. Enzymes remove fibrin deposition and immune complex deposition which are found in inflammatory states. They also promote oxygenation in inflamed tissues. In Europe, systemic enzyme therapies are often used as a first-line agent for treating many inflammatory conditions. My clinical experience has clearly shown the marked benefit that systemic enzymes have in treating all inflammatory conditions. An enzyme is a catalyst—it causes or accelerates a chemical reaction. Enzymes are produced from the basic building blocks in our bodies--amino acids. The human body has over 3,000 enzymes that catalyze over 7,000 enzymatic reactions. Life itself is not possible without an adequate production of enzymes in our body.

Conventional medicine uses enzyme therapies in a wide variety of areas. For example, enzymes are used to break up a blood clot during an acute myocardial infarction (heart attack) or stroke. This therapy is known as thrombolysis.

Enzymes can be thought of as nature's cleaning agents. They help remove debris from injured tissue and send signals to the body that repair needs to begin. When there is insufficient production of enzymes, the healing process is slowed. Taking oral systemic enzymes can aid this healing process, sometimes dramatically.

One of the most amazing systemic enzyme supplements that I have seen for treating inflammatory problems is serrapeptase. Serrapeptase is a proteolytic (breaks down protein) enzyme. Serrapeptase has been shown to be a potent anti-inflammatory agent. Research has shown that serrapeptase induces fibrinolytic (breaks down fibrin) and other anti-inflammatory activity in a number of tissues. [42] [43] As a natural anti-inflammatory agent, serapeptase has shown many positive effects in my patients.

In order to have a systemic effect in the body, enzymes must be taken without food. Furthermore, they must be in enteric coated capsules in order to help the enzymes bypass the stomach. Vitalzyme X®, a serrapeptase enzyme supplement, has proven to be an effective natural anti-inflammatory agent. Another enzyme, Exclzyme 2AF has also proven to be a very effective anti-inflammatory agent.

The only side effects I have noticed with enzymes are occasionally an upset stomach.

RECOMMENDATIONS: For a safe and effective anti-inflammatory effect, it is difficult to beat systemic enzyme therapies. I suggest taking three capsules two to three times per day, without food. Wait at least one hour before eating and at least two hours after eating before ingesting an enzyme supplement. If you take a systemic enzyme capsule with a meal, it will aid in the digestion process but will have little effect as an anti-inflammatory agent. Both enzymes mentioned above can be purchased at my office: www.centerforholisticmedicine.com or by calling 1.866.877.6467).

VITAMIN C

Vitamin C is the most important water soluble antioxidant. Humans are unable to make Vitamin C in their bodies. Therefore, we have to get Vitamin C from our food or supplements. Vitamin C protects proteins and lipids from free radicals that can damage cells and cause chronic illnesses and inflammation. Replenishing Vitamin C levels can have a profound anti-inflammatory effect. I have found it nearly impossible to control or overcome an inflammatory illness without the use of supplemental Vitamin C.

RECOMMENDATIONS: The dose of Vitamin C can vary between individuals. In an acute inflammatory condition, using I.V. Vitamin C is a more efficacious way to increase Vitamin C levels. Orally, I suggest taking from 3-5,000mg of Vitamin C/day. If you get diarrhea, you may need to lower the dose. With an acute inflammatory condition or illness, you may need higher doses of Vitamin C.

GOOD HYDRATION

One of the simplest and most inexpensive methods to promote an anti-inflammatory environment is to drink adequate amounts of water. My clinical experience has shown that dehydration is a major cause of inflammation. Dehydration is caused by inadequate intake of water coupled with the overuse of caffeinated products. Coffee and soda contain caffeine and other substances that have a diuretic effect in the body. In my experience, nothing is more inflammatory to the body than maintaining a dehydrated state. Early morning stiffness is a cardinal sign of dehydration. Our body is 70% water and the brain is 80% water. Drinking adequate amounts of water is the first thing you should do to begin a healthier lifestyle. How much water should you drink? Table 6 below will show you how much water you should drink.

TABLE 6: HOW MUCH WATER SHOULD YOU DRINK?

1. Take your weight in pounds
2. Divide your weight in pounds by 2
3. The resultant number is the amount of water you should ingest in ounces

---

If you are drinking adequate amounts of water, an adequate intake of unrefined salt is necessary for the body. I recommend taking ¼ tsp of unrefined salt for every quart of water ingested. For more information on unrefined salt, I refer the reader to ***Salt Your Way To Health.***

FINAL THOUGHTS

NSAID's have been some of the most profitable drugs for Big Pharma. NSAID's do not treat the underlying cause of any condition. They only treat the symptoms of inflammation. Because they do not treat the underlying cause(s) of an illness, I feel their use should be limited.

The best results for NSAID's occur with short-term use--less than three weeks. In fact, it is unclear if there is any pain-relief benefit from taking NSAID's longer than three weeks. Researchers reported that the pain-relief benefits from NSAID's were limited to the first 2-3 weeks of treatment. After that time period, there was literally no difference between an NSAID and a placebo at providing pain relief in treating inflammation from osteoarthritis. The researchers concluded, "In view of the widespread use of pharmacological agents in {osteoarthritis} management, a discussion is needed to clarify if the limited benefits and considerable costs can justify current recommendations." [44]

Serious adverse effects are associated with all NSAID's including gastrointestinal bleeding and stroke. The natural alternatives reviewed in this chapter are much safer and more cost-effective. These natural agents should be the first line treatment for inflammation while the underlying cause of the inflammation is investigated.

Inflammation in the body can be caused and accelerated by eating a poor diet. Eliminating the use of refined foods and substituting whole foods as well as drinking adequate amounts of water have a marked positive effect on decreasing inflammation. More information about how to improve your diet can be found in ***The Guide to Healthy Eating.***

[1] Laine, L. Approaches to nonsteroidal anti-inflammatory drug use in the high-risk patient. Gastroent. 2001;120:594-606

[2] Singh, G. Epidemiology of NSAID induced gastrointestinal complications. J. Rheum. Suppl. 1999;56:18-24

[3] Wassef, F. Inflammatory modulators. J. of Int. Med. Vol. 1, No. 1. Jan/Feb. 1999

[4] Wolfe, M. Gastrointestinal toxicity of nonsteroidal anti-inflammatory drugs. N. Eng. J. Med. 1999;340:1888-1899

[5] Spiegal, B. Minimizing complications from nonsteroidal anti-inflammatory drugs: cost-effectiveness of competing strategies in varying risk groups. Arthritis Rheum. 2005;53:185-97

[6] Bombardeir, C. Comparison of upper gastrointestinal toxicity of Rofecoxib and naproxen in patients with rheumatoid arthritis. VIGOR study Group. N. Engl. J. Med. 2000;343;1520-8

[7] JAMA. 2000.284:1247-1255

[8] Lancet. 2004;364:665-74

[9] Smalley, W. Nonsteroidal anti-inflammatory drugs and incidence of hospitalizations for peptic ulcer disease in elderly persons. AM. J. Epid. 10995;141:539-545

[10] Lanas. A. Upper gastrointestinal events associated with rofecoxib in a colorectal adenoma chemoprevention trial. Gastoent. 2005. ;129;371

[11] Chan, F. Celecoxib versus diclofenac and omepraczole in reducing the risk of recurrent ulcer bleeding in patients with arthritis. N. Eng. J. Med. 2002;347:2104-2110

[12] Silvestein, F. Gastrointestinal toxicity with celecoxib vs. nonsteroidal anti-inflammatory drugs for osteoarthritis and rheumatoid arthritis: the CLASS study: A randomized controlled trial. Celecoxib long-term arthritis safety study. JAMA. 2000;284:1247-55

[13] Cheng, Y. Role of prostacyclin in the cardiovascular response to thromboxane A2. Science. 20032. Apr. 19;296(5567):539-41

[14] Curr. Chem. Med. 2004. May;11(10):1243-52

[15] Zingjing, A. Adverse effects of cyclooxygenase 2 inhibitors on renal and arrhythmia events. JAMA. Oct. 4, 2006. Vol. 296, No. 13. p. 1619

[16] Harris, R. Physiological regulation of cycooxygenase-2 in the kidney. Am. J. Physiol. Renal. Physiol. 2001;281:F1-F11

[17] Palmer,B . Renal complications associated with the use of non-steroidal anti-inflammatory agents. J. Investig. Med. 1995;43:516-533

[18] Scholondorff, D. Renal complications of non-steoidal anti-inflammatory drugs. Kidney Intl. 1993:44:643-653

[19] Annals of Int. Medicine. 2000;133:1-9.

[20] Hippisley-Cox, J. Risk of myocardial infarction in patiatns taking cyclooxygenase-2 inhibitors or conventional non-steoridal anti-inflammaotry drugs: populiaton based nested case-control analysis. BMJ. (11 June). 330.7504.1366

[21] Ulinski, T. Renal complications of non-steroidal anti-inflammaries. Arch. Pediat. 2004l. Jul;11(7)885-8

[22] ULinski, T. Acute renal failure after treatment with non-steroidal anti-inflammatory drugs. Eur. J. Pediatr. 2004. Mar;163(3):148-50

[23] Perniger, TV. Risk of kidney failure associated with the use of acetaminophen, aspirin and nonsteroidal anti-inflammatory drugs. N. Eng. J. Med. 1994. Dec 22:331(25):1675-9

[24] Perna, A. Increased plasma protein homocysteinylation in hemodialsys pateitns. Kidney Int. 2006. Mar;69(5):869-76

[25] Tsai, JC. Correlation of plasma homocysteine level with arterial stiffnes an pulse pressure in hemodialysis patients. Atherosclerosis. 2005. Set;182(1):121-7

[26] Bombardier, C. IBID. 2000

[27] Bombardeir, C. IBID. 2000

[28] Los Angeles Times. Oct. 11, 2004

[29] Rubin, Rita. How did the Vioxx debacle happen. USA Today. 10.12.2004

[30] Rubin, Rita. IBID. 2004

[31] Interview of Dr. David Graham in The Crusader. June/July 2005.

[32] Life Extension Magazine. February, 2005.

[33] Interview of Dr. David Graham. IBID. 2005

[34] Wassef, Farid. Inflammatory Modulators. International Journal of Integrative Medicine. Vol. 1, No. 1. Jan/Feb. 1999

[35] FDA Consumer Magazine. Nov.- Dec. 2004 issue. FDA.gov/fdac/features/2004/604

[36] Mayatepek, E. Influence of dietary (n-3)-polyunsaturated fatty acids on leukotriene B4 and prostaglandin E2 synthesis and course of experimental tuberculosis in guinea pigs. Infecton. 1994. Mar;22(2):106-12

[37] Stammers T, Sibblad B, Freeling P. Fish oil in osteoarthritis. Lancet. 1989. Aug 26;2(8661):503.

[38] Hagfors L, Nilsson I, Skoldstam L, Johansson G. Fat intake and composition of fatty acids in serum phospholipids in a randomized, controlled, Mediterranean dietary intervention study on patients with rheumatoid arthritis. Nutr. Metab. (Lond). 2005 Oct 10;2:26.

[39] Volker D, Fitzgerald P, Major G, Gang M. Efficacy of fish oil concentrate in the treatment of rheumatoid arthritis. J. Rheumatol. 2000 Oct;27(10):2343-6.

[40] James MJ, Cleland LG. Dietary n-3 fatty acids and therapy for rheumatoid arthritis. Semin Arthritis Rheum. 1997 Oct;27(2):85-97.

[41] Nakamura, H. Effects of glucosamine administration on patients with rheumatoid arthritis. Rheumatol. Int. 2006. Sep. 5. EPub ahead of print.

[42] Mazone, A. Evaluation of Serratia peptidase in acute or chronic inflammation of otorhinolaryngology pathology: a multicentre, double-blind randomized trial versus placebo. J. Int. Med. Res. 1990;18(5):379-88

[43] Esch, PM. Reduction of postoperative swelling. Objective measurement to swelling of the upper ankle joint in treatment with serapeptase-a prospective study. Fortschr. Med. 19890;107(4):67-8

[44] Eur. J. Pain. 2006. M ay 6;DOI:10.1016/J.ejpain. 2006.02.013

Chapter 9

Hormone Replacement Therapy

INTRODUCTION

For over 25 years, the media and nearly all mainstream medical organizations promoted the use of conventional hormone replacement therapy (HRT) as the miracle medical treatment. Conventional HRT was touted as an effective regimen for treating menopausal symptoms, cardiovascular disease, and osteoporosis.

During this time, there were headlines in the newspapers which consistently pointed to the positive effects of conventional HRT therapy.   Doctors went to conferences sponsored by Big Pharma informing them that nearly every woman could benefit from conventional HRT therapy.   The lead articles in the most prestigious medical journals reported on the benefits of conventional hormones.   Anyone questioning the use of conventional HRT therapy was roundly criticized.

However, when the truth finally became apparent to all, the use of synthetic hormones did not look so good. In fact, these foreign substances were found to cause a lot of serious adverse effects such as breast cancer, heart attacks, and strokes. How could so many intelligent people be so wrong? Why were women misled for over 25 years?

The answer to these questions can be found in a statement I made at the beginning of this book; **you can't poison a crucial enzyme or block an important receptor for the long-term and expect a good result.** Conventional HRT uses synthetic, foreign hormones that block our bodies' normal hormonal receptors and cause many serious adverse effects. On the other hand, our bodies have receptors for binding natural, bioidentical hormones. These topics will be explained throughout this chapter.

WHAT IS THE DIFFERENCE BETWEEN SYNTHETIC AND BIOIDENTICAL HORMONES?

A hormone is a chemical substance produced in the body by a gland. Hormones have a specific regulatory effect on the activity of the body. For example, the thyroid gland produces thyroid hormone which helps to regulate the metabolism of the body.

Bioidentical, natural hormones are substances generally produced from plant products that closely mimic the body's own hormone production, both structurally and chemically. Examples of bioidentical hormones include: DHEA, natural progesterone, natural estrogens, natural testosterone, melatonin, hydrocortisone, human growth hormone, and pregnenolone. Hormones that have been chemically altered are termed synthetic hormones.

Synthetic hormones are not naturally occurring substances in the body. In fact, synthetic hormones are not found in any living forms. Synthetic hormones can therefore be thought of as foreign substances to the body. Because they are foreign substances to the body, is there any wonder that there are so many serious side effects with the use of synthetic hormones? Examples of synthetic hormones include Provera®, Prempro®, Premarin®, birth control pills, etc.

THE LOCK AND KEY MODEL OF HORMONES

All of the hormones in our bodies work via a "lock and key"' model. When a hormone is released from its gland the hormone (the "key") binds to its receptor (the "lock"). This binding is analogous to a key being put in the ignition of the car. When the hormone binds to its receptor, a chemical reaction takes place. Natural, bioidentical hormones have a perfect fit in these receptors. The "key" fits perfectly in its complimentary "lock". This is contrasted with a synthetic hormone in which the unnatural hormone (i.e., the wrong "key") does not fit well in the body's receptor (i.e., the "lock").

A comparison of the chemical structure of a natural hormone (progesterone) and a synthetic hormone (Provera®) is shown in Figure 1. Provera® is the synthetic version of the hormone progesterone. As can be seen from Figure 1, Provera® has two side chains (indicated by arrows) that progesterone does not have. These side chains make Provera® a foreign substance to the body.

Figure 1: A Comparison of a Bioidentical Hormone (Progesterone) and a Synthetic Hormone (Provera®)

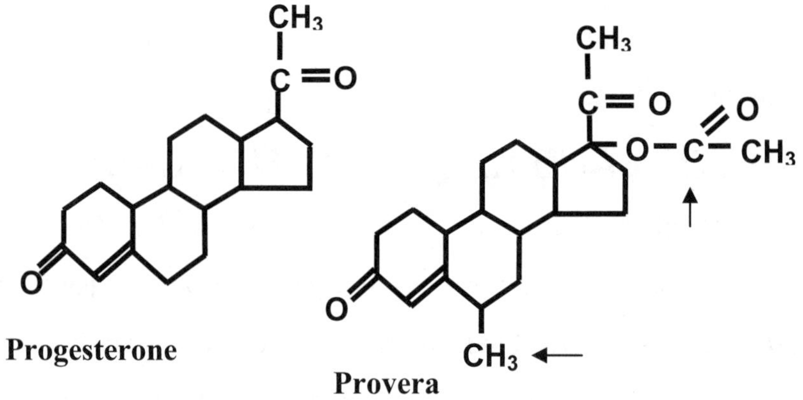

Progesterone

Provera

The difference between the natural bioidentical hormone, progesterone, and the synthetic version, Provera®, is illustrated in this diagram. The arrows in the Provera® illustration point out the additional side chains added to progesterone. These added chains make Provera® a foreign substance in the body, leading to an increased risk of adverse effects.

The reason there are so many adverse effects with conventional HRT is because the body does not have receptors for these unnatural hormones to bind to. For example, when the synthetic hormone Provera® binds to the receptor for progesterone, Provera® will not fit correctly in that receptor. This poor fit is responsible for the adverse effects of Provera® which are described further in this chapter.

I believe that if we are going to use a hormone to treat any condition, we should use a natural, bioidentical hormone over a synthetic hormone every time.

WHY WOULD SYNTHETIC HORMONES BE PRODUCED?

Let's take a closer look at Figure 1. When you look at the difference between the chemical structures of progesterone and Provera®, a question comes to mind; why would Big Pharma alter progesterone by putting those side chains (indicated by the arrows in Figure 1) on progesterone? The answer is: to develop a patentable product that can maximize profits.

Natural substances cannot be patented. For example, Vitamin C or magnesium cannot be patented. However, a foreign substance can be patented. Big Pharma's job is to maximize profits for its shareholders. It is much more profitable to promote a patented product than it is to promote a natural product. Remember, anyone can manufacture and promote Vitamin C.

Only the company that holds the patent to a foreign substance such as Provera® can manufacture and promote it.

PROVERA®

Provera® is the synthetic version of the hormone progesterone. Provera® contains two side chains indicated by arrows in Figure 1 that the hormone progesterone does not have. These side chains make Provera® an unnatural substance for the human body.

According The Physicians Desk Reference (PDR), Provera® is indicated for the:

1. Reduction of endometrial hyperplasia in post-menopausal women taking estrogens
2. Treatment of abnormal uterine bleeding due to hormonal imbalance in the absence of organic pathology
3. Prevention of pregnancy
4. Initiation of menses when amenorrhea is present

With the exception of preventing pregnancy, all of the above indications can be managed by the bioidentical hormone progesterone without the serious adverse effects caused by Provera®.

ADVERSE EFFECTS OF PROVERA®:
IRREVERSIBLE OSTEOPOROSIS

Provera®, being a synthetic agent, is associated with multiple side effects. As previously mentioned, for over 25 years, women were assured by main-stream medical organizations that synthetic HRT was safe. However, the research showed otherwise.

Provera® has been shown to cause irreversible osteoporosis. It has been given a 'black-box' warning from the FDA stating, "Women who use Depo-Provera® may experience a significant decrease in bone mineral density that might not be completely reversible after discontinuing use."[1] How could the use of one drug cause irreversible osteoporosis? It goes back to the statement that *you can't poison a crucial enzyme or block an important receptor for the long-term and expect a good result.* Provera®, being a foreign substance to the body, blocks the body's receptors for progesterone. Furthermore, since it is a foreign substance, the body has a difficult time detoxifying Provera®. The end result is a whole host of serious adverse effects such as irreversible osteoporosis. Instead of putting Depo-Provera in the 'black box', the FDA should remove it from the market. I don't believe anyone should use Provera for any condition, especially when there is a natural, bioidentical form of progesterone readily available.

ADVERSE EFFECTS OF PROVERA®: THE WOMEN'S HEALTH INITIATIVE

The most publicized research study involving HRT was the Women's Health Initiative. The Women's Health Initiative (WHI) was designed to provide information about the risks and benefits of conventional hormone replacement therapy. The WHI was a study involving 40 large medical centers around the United States, with 16,608 women. The WHI began in 1996 and was reported in July, 2002.

The WHI was a randomized, placebo-controlled study. This means that half of the women received conventional hormone replacement in the form of Prempro® (Premarin® and Provera®) and half received a placebo (no active drug).

The outcomes the researchers were looking for included increases or decreases in breast cancer, heart disease, stroke, pulmonary embolism, colorectal cancer, endometrial cancer, hip fracture, and death due to any cause.

The study was supposed to last 8.5 years. The researchers halted the study at 5.2 years because the overall risks of conventional hormone replacement therapy outweighed the overall benefits.

FIGURE 1: RESULTS OF WHI

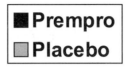

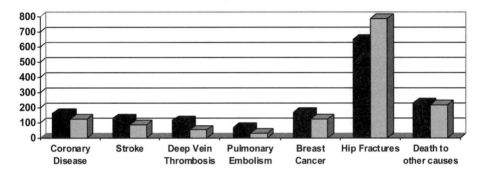

Results of WHI: The Good

Figure 1 shows the results of the WHI. There were positive outcomes reported from WHI. There was a 21% decrease in osteoporotic fractures in the Prempro® group as compared to the placebo group. In addition, there was a 37% decrease in colorectal cancer in the Prempro® group.

Results of WHI: The Bad

There was a 29% increase in coronary heart disease in the Prempro® group.

Results of WHI: The Ugly

A 41% increase in stroke and a remarkable 2,100% increase in pulmonary embolism (i.e., lung blood clots) was found in the treated (i.e., Prempro®) group. In addition the Prempro® group had a 26% increased risk of breast cancer.

The Implications of WHI

The WHI was supposed to be an 8.5-year study. However, the research was stopped early, at 5.2 years, when the authors of the study realized that the risks of conventional hormone replacement therapy outweighed the benefits.

The results of the WHI made national headlines. It was the final blow to the widespread use of conventional hormone replacement therapy. Women were flocking to their doctors asking them what to do with their hormone replacement therapy. The headlines in the newspapers across the country suggested that important, new information had come to light on the use of conventional hormones.

Since the WHI made such an impact nationwide, the question to ask is: What were the new findings in the WHI that made so many women and their physicians question the benefits of taking conventional hormone replacement therapy?

The answer to the above question can be summed up in one word: **nothing**. There was no new information in the WHI that wasn't already available in the past. In fact, many other studies had already shown the negative influences conventional hormone replacement therapy had on cardiovascular disease, strokes, and other blood clots as well as cancer. However, this information was only available to those who carefully read these research reports. Reading the abstracts from these studies would not provide their true outcomes. The media often only parrots what Big Pharma wants them to report from these studies. Let's take a closer look at what some of these studies actually did show.

Coronary Artery Disease

For over 25 years, Big Pharma assured women that conventional HRT would protect them from heart disease. However, the research did not support this claim. Many studies found an increased risk of heart disease caused by conventional HRT. The increased risk for cardiac events associated with conventional hormone replacement therapy has been reported in many different studies.

In a landmark article in 1998, researchers reported increased cardiovascular events in the conventional hormone-treated group as compared to a controlled group that took a placebo.[2] The American Heart Association came out against using conventional hormone replacement therapy for the sole reason of preventing future heart attacks.[3] An article in the New

England Journal of Medicine cited similar results showing conventional hormone replacement therapy ineffective for preventing heart disease.[4]

The Women's Health Initiative research study showed a 29% increase in cardiovascular disease in the group that took Prempro®. This study confirmed the earlier studies on the ineffectiveness of conventional hormone replacement therapy in preventing cardiovascular disease.

In addition, WHI showed that there was no benefit for stroke prevention. Instead, women who took conventional hormones had a 41% increased risk of stroke compared to women who did not take the hormones. It is even more alarming that a 2,100% increased risk for pulmonary embolism was observed.

Breast Cancer

Perhaps the greatest downfall of conventional HRT was the finding that it caused an increased risk of breast cancer. The concern with increasing the risk for breast cancer by using conventional hormones has been around for over 25 years. Many previous studies have shown an increased risk of breast cancer with the use of conventional hormones.[5][6][7][8].

Breast cancer is every woman's fear. It is occurring at epidemic rates in this country. Today, approximately one in seven women in the United States is affected by breast cancer.

With such high rates of breast cancer prevalent today, no therapy should be prescribed that further increases the rate of breast cancer. The WHI clearly showed that the use of conventional hormones was responsible for a 26% increased risk of breast cancer. As mentioned above, the WHI was not the first study to point out this increased risk. The studies showing an increased risk of breast cancer date back to the early 1980's. This information was not widely publicized because it would have resulted in a dramatic decline in the use of these synthetic hormones.

As a physician, I took an oath at my medical school graduation that said in part, "Above all, do no harm". The WHI study, as well as many previous studies, showed that the use of conventional, synthetic hormones is often harmful. I believe safer methods need to be examined, and this will only occur with the use of bio-identical (i.e., natural) hormones. Synthetic hormones have no place in anybody's regimen.

PROGESTERONE

The hormone progesterone, as pictured in Figure 1, is produced in the adrenal glands of both men and women. Furthermore, the ovaries produce significant amounts of progesterone. Because the body has specific receptors for progesterone, it has mechanisms to properly bind and detoxify progesterone. Bioidentical progesterone should be the only form of progesterone used. Synthetic forms should never be used.

The benefits of bioidentical progesterone are varied. Progesterone is a safe and effective treatment for a variety of conditions including: fibrocystic breast disease, menopausal symptoms, PMS, and endometriosis. It has also been shown to:

1. Function as a natural antidepressant
2. Facilitate thyroid function
3. Improve blood sugar
4. Improve cell oxygenation
5. Function as a natural diuretic

Unlike bioidentical progesterone, Provera® does not have any of these five positive attributes as listed for progesterone. Furthermore, Provera® does not treat any of the conditions mentioned above. When should Provera® ever be used? The answer to this question is that Provera® should never be used for any condition. Provera® is a toxic substance to the body and has no place in any medical therapy.

For more information on the benefits and uses of natural, bioidentical progesterone, I refer the reader to ***The Miracle of Natural Hormones, 3rd Edition.***

PROVERA® VERSUS PROGESTERONE

Why would Provera® not have any of the positive effects that progesterone has in the body? Why would Provera® have so many adverse effects associated with its use? Figure 1 shows us the answer. Provera®, having those two side chains inserted into the progesterone molecule, is a foreign substance to the body. When Provera® is taken, it will bind to the receptors for progesterone.   This binding process blocks the progesterone receptor from binding progesterone.   It effectively makes the body deficient in progesterone. This deficiency of progesterone, coupled with the blocking of its receptors is responsible for all of the serious adverse effects from Provera®.

The use of a synthetic progesterone derivative such as Provera® provides the body with two major problems:

1.   Provera® binds to the progesterone receptor. This makes the receptor unable to bind progesterone and leads to a progesterone deficiency.

2.   Being a foreign substance in the body, there are no adequate detoxifying mechanisms for the body to release Provera® from its binding. This causes Provera® to stay in the body much too long and exacerbates the adverse effects.

SHOULD ANYONE TAKE PROVERA®?

Provera®, like all synthetic, foreign hormones is associated with a myriad of adverse effects. The mechanism of these substances causing adverse effects is the same: *by poisoning crucial enzymes and blocking important receptors, adverse effects are bound to occur.* There is no reason to use a synthetic hormone for any condition when there are natural, bioidentical versions available. As previously stated, I do not believe Provera® should ever be used for any condition.

WHY USE BIOIDENTICAL, NATURAL HORMONES?

Bioidentical, natural hormones, when used appropriately, will enhance one's health and will treat or even cure diseases, all without any appreciable side effects. Many physicians erroneously believe there is no difference between a synthetic hormone and a bioidentical, natural hormone. That is usually because these physicians have little or no experience in the use of bioidentical natural hormones and other natural products. My clinical experience shows that there is no better substitute for the body's own production of hormones than the use of a natural form of that hormone. This experience has been repeatedly confirmed by my patients' positive responses to natural hormones.

Natural hormones can improve well-being, slow aging, and reverse many chronic conditions. After taking natural hormones, my older patients constantly proclaim that they feel like they did when they were in their 20's. I have found natural hormones to be a great benefit and often a cure for many conditions including chronic fatigue syndrome, PMS, endometriosis, infertility, headaches and migraine headaches, recurrent infections, fibromyalgia, ulcerative colitis, Crohn's, and other autoimmune disorders. It is rare for patients with any of the above conditions not to show significant improvement in their conditions after balancing the hormonal system with natural, bioidentical hormones. I am continually amazed at how many chronic diseases can be halted and, many times, cured through the use of natural, bioidentical hormones.

Man has searched for a fountain of youth for thousands of years. Although there is no "cure" for aging, my clinical experience has shown that natural hormones, when used appropriately, can slow down many of the signs of aging including deteriorating mental function, loss of muscle tone, and wrinkled skin. Hormone production peaks when we are young, usually in the age range from 20 to 30. In older people, supplementation with natural, bioidentical hormones can reverse many of the signs of aging. Synthetic hormones do not provide the same anti-aging benefits as natural, bioidentical hormones.

My patients are familiar with the following question: "If it is found that you are low in a hormone, and you are given a choice of a natural, bioidentical hormone—one that closely mimics your own hormone chemically and structurally, versus a synthetic hormone—a man-made derivative of a hormone that has been structurally altered to become a patentable product, which one would you pick?" A vast scientific knowledge base is not needed to realize a natural, bioidentical hormone will perform better than a synthetic hormone every time. This statement holds true when comparing all natural products to synthetic products, including vitamins, minerals, and herbs. It is a common-sense argument to use a natural product over a foreign substance to treat disease and promote health, and there are multiple studies that back up this idea.

FINAL THOUGHTS

When there are bioidentical, natural versions of a hormone available, the synthetic versions should not be used. Provera®, the synthetic version of progesterone (see Figure 1) should never be used. Its use is associated with many serious adverse effects including an increased risk of breast cancer, heart attacks, stroke, and irreversible osteoporosis. Provera® does not treat any condition caused by a hormonal imbalance; it actually causes a hormonal imbalance. By blocking the receptor for progesterone, it causes a progesterone deficiency. When there is a progesterone deficiency present, bioidentical progesterone should be the treatment of choice. The same argument holds for estrogens—Premarin should never be used (unless you are treating a pregnant horse). When estrogen therapy is indicated, natural, bioidentical estrogens should be used. For more information about bioidentical hormones I refer the reader to ***The Miracle of Natural Hormones, 3rd Edition.***

While the first edition of this book was in publication, researchers from the M.D. Anderson Cancer Center reported that in the U.S., rates of the most common form of breast cancer dropped 15% from August 2002 to December 2003. Researchers have speculated that the decline may be due to women stopping their use of synthetic hormones after the Women's Health Initiative was released in the July of 2002.[9] A second study reported in November, 2006 showed that breast cancer rates in California also fell during the same time period.[10]

Big Pharma tried to downplay the dropping breast cancer rate by claiming that since the WHI, women were getting less mammograms. Well, this was proven untrue as the mammogram rate was virtually unchanged.

A recent study in the New England Journal of Medicine found that there was a 26% increase in breast cancer for those women who took conventional HRT (Premarin and Provera) during the length of the study. [11]

A follow-up analysis found that when the women were told to stop the synthetic hormones, the breast cancer rate declined by 26% over the following 2.5 years.

The post-analysis of the WHI showing a declining breast cancer rate when women stop taking synthetic hormones truly shows the danger of conventional hormone replacement therapy. These foreign substances need to be avoided.

Finally, it makes common sense that no synthetic hormone should be used for any condition when there is a bioidentical, natural version of the hormone available. Looking at physiology and biochemistry it becomes clear that using a synthetic, foreign hormone in the body is bound to cause trouble. My clinical experience has clearly shown the benefits of balancing the hormonal system with bioidentical natural hormones.

[1] FP News. 01.2005

[2] Hulley, Stephen, et al. Randomized trial of estrogen plus progestin for secondary prevention of coronary heart disease in postmenopausal women. JAMA. Vol. 280 No. 7, 8/19/98

[3] Circulation. July 24, 2001;104;459-503

[4] New England Journal of Medicine. 8/24/00;343:522-529

[5] J. Natl. Cancer Inst. 92(4) 328-332, 2000

[6] Menopausal Estrogen and Estrogen-Progestin Replacement Therapy and Breast Cancer Risk. JAMA. 1/26/2000. Vol. 283, No.4

[7] The risk of breast cancer after estrogen and estrogen-progestin replacement. N. Engl. J. Med. 1989;321:293-297

[8] The use of estrogens and progestins and the risk of breast cancer in postmenopausal women. N. Engl. J. Med. 1995;332:1589-1593

[9] New York Times. 12.15.2006 and Wall Street Journal 12.15.2006

[10] Clarke, Christina. Recent declines in hormone therapy utilization and breast cacner incidence: Clinical and population-based evidence. Correspondence. Journal of Clinical Oncology. Vol. 24. N. 33. Nov. 20, 2006

[11] NEJM. 2.5.09. Vol. 360;6:673.

Chapter 10

Final Thoughts

FINAL THOUGHTS

It has been two years since I wrote the first edition of *Drugs That Don't Work and Natural Therapies That Do.* Since that time, our use of prescription drugs has only increased. As we try to reform our health care system we should keep in mind what we are trying to achieve. If we are trying to achieve a healthier society, I am afraid we are going down the wrong path. The diabetes epidemic as described in chapter 4 is an example of what is wrong. Instead of focusing on the underlying problem causing this epidemic (poor lifestyle choices), conventional medicine is focused on ineffective drug therapies.

The National Center for Health Statistics reported that between 1997 and 2002 expenses for prescription drugs increased 75%. Since then, this trend has only continued to increase. Approximately 45% of Americans use at least one prescription drug.[1][2] The Kaiser Family Foundation reports 2.1 billion prescriptions were written in 1994 and 3.5 billion prescriptions were written in 2004—a 68% increase. Spending for U.S. prescription drugs was 188.5 billion dollars in 2004, a 450% increase since 1990.[3] Unbelievably, it is projected that in 2015, prescription drug spending will exceed 446.2 billion dollars.

We spend more money on health care than any other country. Are we healthier for this increased use in prescription medications? The answer is unequivocally "no".

In almost every health parameter measured, the United States lags behind other western countries. In fact, over the last 30 years, the United States has fallen further behind the other western countries in nearly every category of health system performance.[4] All during this time, the U.S. was outspending every other country on health care.

Our medical system is broken. It is a system based on the disease and drug model. Physicians are trained to properly diagnose the illness and to prescribe the drug therapy to treat the symptoms of the illness. Physicians are not educated about wellness or about how to help patients achieve their optimal health.

Drugs do not promote health. In most cases, they only modify the symptoms of a disease process. The drugs, via blocking receptors or poisoning enzymes, often have harmful side effects that cannot be predicted in the individual.

This book was written to educate the reader about the mechanism of how the most common drugs work in the body. If the public were more educated about what these drugs do in our bodies, I think they would be less likely to take the drugs and more likely to search for safe and effective alternatives.

Prescription drug use does have its place. In an emergent condition, drugs can be lifesaving. However, the long-term use of drugs is fraught with adverse effects. Physicians should not be so quick to prescribe a drug if there is a natural alternative available. I have seen many illnesses improve without the use of drugs.

In order to achieve our optimal health, we need to supply the body with the basic raw materials that it needs. Drugs are not part of those raw materials. Eating a healthy diet, drinking water, exercising, and detoxifying, are examples of ways to improve your health. I have written seven books to help get this message out.

You can make changes in your lifestyle which will positively impact your overall health. Educate yourself about a drug therapy before you take it. If the mechanism of action of the drug doesn't make sense, search for an alternative. Remember, prescription drugs generally block important receptors or poison crucial enzymes. We should strive to enhance physiology and biochemistry, not disrupt it. The sole reliance on drug therapies doesn't make sense in most cases. I hope this book gets everyone looking for safer alternatives to drug therapies.

TO ALL OF OUR HEALTH!

[1] From CDC.gov
[2] WSOCTV.com
[3] Kaiser Family Foundation. Prescription drug trends fact sheet. June 2006
[4] Anderson, G. Health Affairs. May/June 2001

Index

A

Achlorhydria 163-165
Aciphex 159
Actonel 133, 135, 142
Adrenal hormones 31-34, 36, 278-299
Anemia, 165
Angina 19
Aspartame 222, 228
Asthma 191-193
Avandia 88
Axid 159

B

Bioidentical hormones 35-37, 96-97, 278-281, 289-296
Bisphosphonates 122, 130-142, 152
Bone mineral density test 114-122, 131-133, 145
Boniva 133, 135
Breast cancer 277, 286, 288-289, 295-296

C

Calcium 107-108, 110, 113, 127, 130, 145, 147-150, 152
Candida 170
C. difficile 168-170, 187
Celiac disease 128-129
Celebrex 249-252, 256
Celexa 202
CoQ10 41, 48-53
Coumadin 126-127
Crestor 47, 63-67

D

DHEA 96, 124, 235, 278

E

Evista 142

F

Fish oil 149, 263
Food allergies 228-230
Fosomax 112, 114, 133-138, 140, 145

G

Gastritis 175-176
GERD 181-186
Glucosamine 266
Gluten 129, 229
Graves' disease 190

H

Hashimoto's disease 190

Heartburn 172-173, 175
Hepatitis 142
HMG-CoA reductase 47-49
H. pylori 163, 166-168, 176-181
Hydrochloric acid 161-163, 165-167, 174-176, 178-179, 181-182, 187-188, 191-193

I

Insulin Resistance 80-82, 92
Iodine 98

L

LDL-cholesterol 54, 57, 64
Lipitor 45, 47-48, 51

M

Magnesium 97, 150

Mastic 179
Metformin 87

N

Nattokinase 151
Nexium 154, 163, 167, 169, 176, 190-191

O

Osteoblasts 108-114, 137, 141
Osteoclasts 108-114, 134-135, 137, 141
Osteogenesis imperfecta 106, 109, 113
Osteonecrosis 140-141
Osteoporosis 103-106, 114-127, 129-133, 138, 142-149, 151-152

P

Pancreatitis 142
Pepcid 159, 170
Pernicious anemia 164
pH 144-145
Pravachol 45-46, 48
Pregnenolone 124, 131
Prevacid 159
Prilosec 159, 162-164, 173, 176, 190
Progesterone 235, 278-283, 289-291, 294
Provera 279-284, 290-292, 294
Prozac 199-200, 212
Protonix 159

R

Ravnskov, Uffe 46, 59
Rheumatoid arthritis 190

S

Sanson, Gillian 117-118, 138, 143
Serotonin 201-202, 204-211, 218, 220-223, 225-226, 228, 231
SSRI's 201-204, 208-214
Statins 28, 46, 48-54, 56, 58, 70

Strontium 149, 152

T

Testosterone 31, 124, 131
Tryptophan 205, 221-224, 226

U

Uveitis 142

V

Vioxx 249-252, 256, 258-260,
Vitamin B12 128, 151, 165
Vitamin C 263, 269
Vitamin D 37, 148-149
Vitamin E 149
Vitamin K 126-129, 190
Vytorin 69-70

W

Women's Health Initiative 284-289

Z

Zantac 174
Zegerid 159
Zinc 146, 149, 107
Zocor 44, 48-49
Zoloft 208
Zometa 135

Books by David Brownstein, M.D.

IODINE: WHY YOU NEED IT, WHY YOU CAN'T LIVE WITHOUT IT, 4th EDITION

Iodine is the most misunderstood nutrient. Dr. Brownstein shows you the benefit of supplementing with iodine. Iodine deficiency is rampant. Iodine deficiency is a world-wide problem and is at near epidemic levels in the United States. Most people wrongly assume that you get enough iodine from iodized salt. Dr. Brownstein convincingly shows you why it is vitally important to get your iodine levels measured. He shows you how iodine deficiency is related to:

- Breast cancer
- Hypothyroidism and Graves' disease
- Autoimmune illnesses
- Chronic Fatigue and Fibromyalgia
- Cancer of the prostate, ovaries and much more!

DRUGS THAT DON'T WORK and NATURAL THERAPIES THAT DO, 2nd Edition

Dr. Brownstein's newest book will show you why the most commonly prescribed drugs may not be your best choice. Dr. Brownstein shows why drugs have so many adverse effects. The following conditions are covered in this book: high cholesterol levels, depression, GERD and reflux esophagitis, osteoporosis, inflammation and hormone imbalances. He also gives examples of natural substances that can help the body heal.

See why the following drugs need to be avoided:

- Cholesterol-lowering drugs (statins such as Lipitor, Zocor, Mevacor, and Crestor and Zetia)
- Antidepressant drugs (SSRI's such as Prozac, Zoloft, Celexa, Paxil)
- Antacid drugs (H-2 blockers and PPI's such as Nexium, Prilosec, and Zantac)
- Osteoporosis drugs (Bisphosphonates such as Fosomax and Actonel, Zometa, and Boniva)
- Diabetes drugs (Metformin, Avandia, Glucotrol, etc.)
- Anti-inflammatory drugs (Celebrex, Vioxx, Motrin, Naprosyn, etc)
- Synthetic Hormones (Provera and Estrogen)

SALT YOUR WAY TO HEALTH, 2nd Edition

Dr. Brownstein dispels many of the myths of salt. Salt is bad for you. Salt causes hypertension. These are just a few of the myths Dr. Brownstein tackles in this book. He shows you how the right kind of salt--unrefined salt--can have a remarkable health benefit to the body. Refined salt is a toxic, devitalized substance for the body. Unrefined salt is a necessary ingredient for achieving your optimal health. See how adding unrefined salt to your diet can help you:

- Maintain a normal blood pressure
- Balance your hormones
- Optimize your immune system
- Lower your risk for heart disease
- Overcome chronic illness

THE MIRACLE OF NATURAL HORMONES, 3RD EDITION

Optimal health cannot be achieved with an imbalanced hormonal system. Dr. Brownstein's research on bioidentical hormones provides the reader with a plethora of information on the benefits of balancing the hormonal system with bioidentical, natural hormones. This book is in its third edition. This book gives actual case studies of the benefits of natural hormones.

See how balancing the hormonal system can help:

- Arthritis and autoimmune disorders
- Chronic fatigue syndrome and fibromyalgia
- Heart disease
- Hypothyroidism
- Menopausal symptoms
- And much more!

OVERCOMING THYROID DISORDERS, 2nd Edition

This book provides new insight into why thyroid disorders are frequently undiagnosed and how best to treat them. The holistic treatment plan outlined in this book will show you how safe and natural remedies can help improve your thyroid function and help you achieve your optimal health. NEW SECOND EDITION!

- Detoxification
- Diet
- Graves'
- Hashimoto's Disease
- Hypothyroidism
- And Much More!!

OVERCOMING ARTHRITIS

Dr. Brownstein shows you how a holistic approach can help you overcome arthritis, fibromyalgia, chronic fatigue syndrome, and other conditions. This approach encompasses the use of:

- Allergy elimination
- Detoxification
- Diet
- Natural, bioidentical hormones
- Vitamins and minerals
- Water

THE GUIDE TO HEALTHY EATING, 2nd Edition

Which food do you buy? Where to shop? How do you prepare food? This book will answer all of these questions and much more. Dr. Brownstein co-wrote this book with his nutritionist, Sheryl Shenefelt, C.N. Eating the healthiest way is the most important thing you can do. This book contains recipes and information on how best to feed your family. See how eating a healthier diet can help you:

- Avoid chronic illness
- Enhance your immune system
- Improve your family's nutrition

THE GUIDE TO A GLUTEN-FREE DIET, 2nd Edition

What would you say if 16% of the population (1/6) had a serious, life-threatening illness that was only being diagnosed correctly only 3% of the time? Gluten-sensitivity is the most frequently missed diagnosis in the U.S. This book will show how you can incorporate a healthier lifestyle by becoming gluten-free.

- Why you should become gluten-free
- What illnesses are associated with gluten sensitivity
- How to shop and cook gluten-free
- Where to find gluten-free resources

The Guide to a Dairy-free Diet

This book will show you why dairy is not a healthy food. Dr. Brownstein and Sheryl Shenefelt, CCN, will provide you the information you need to become dairy free. This book will dispel the myth that dairy from pasteurized milk is a healthy food choice. In fact, it is a devitalized food source which needs to be avoided.

Read this book to see why common dairy foods including milk cause:

- Osteoporosis
- Diabetes
- Allergies
- Asthma
- A Poor Immune System

The Soy Deception

This book will dispel the myths of soy being a healthy food. Soy ingestion can cause a myriad of severe health issues. Read this book to see why soy can cause:

- Allergies
- Cancer
- Osteoporosis
- Thyroid Disorders
- A Poor Immune System
- And, Much More!

Call 1-888-647-5616 or send a check or money order
BOOKS $15 each!

Sales Tax: For Michigan residents, please add $.90 per book.

Shipping :	1-3 Books	$5.00
	4-6 Books:	$4.00
	7-9 Books:	$3.00
	10 Books:	FREE SHIPPING!

VOLUME DISCOUNTS AVAILABLE. CALL 1-888-647-5616 FOR MORE
DVD's of Dr. Brownstein's Latest Lectures Available!
INFORMATION OR ORDER ON-LINE AT: WWW.DRBROWNSTEIN.COM
You can send a check to: **Medical Alternatives Press**
                            4173 Fieldbrook
                            West Bloomfield, MI 48323